WHJ 1207

Books should be returned to the SDH Library on or before
the date stamped above unless a renewal has been arranged.

SALISBURY DISTRICT HOS
Tel: Salisbury 336262
Out of hours answer mach

The Audit Handbook

The Audit Handbook

Improving Health Care through Clinical Audit

I.K. CROMBIE
H.T.O. DAVIES
S.C.S. ABRAHAM
C. DU V. FLOREY

University of Dundee,
Ninewells Hospital and Medical School, Dundee

JOHN WILEY & SONS
Chichester · New York · Brisbane · Toronto · Singapore

Other Wiley Editorial Offices

John Wiley & Sons, Inc., 605 Third Avenue,
New York, NY 10158-0012, USA

Jacaranda Wiley Ltd, 33 Park Road, Milton,
Queensland 4064, Australia

John Wiley & Sons (Canada) Ltd, 22 Worcester Road,
Rexdale, Ontario M9W 1L1, Canada

John Wiley & Sons (SEA) Pte Ltd, 37 Jalan Pemimpin #05-04,
Block B, Union Industrial Building, Singapore 2057

Library of Congress Cataloging-in-Publication Data

The Audit handbook : improving health care through clinical audit /
  I. K. Crombie ... [et al.].
    p. cm.
  Includes bibliographical references and index.
  ISBN 0 471 93766 5
  1. Medical audit. I. Crombie, I. K.
  [DNLM: 1. Medical Audit—Great Britain. W 84 FA1 A9 1993]
RA399.A1A93 1993
362.1'068—dc20
DNLM/DLC
for Library of Congress   92-48371
                                        CIP

British Library Cataloguing in Publication Data

A catalogue record for this book is available from the British Library

ISBN 0 471 93766 5

Typeset in 11/13pt Palatino from author's disks by Text Processing Department,
John Wiley & Sons Ltd, Chichester
Printed and bound in Great Britain by
Biddles Ltd, Guildford and King's Lynn

To Mum and Dad, and Jean—IC

To my mother and father, and to Catherine—HD

Contents

Preface

Audit has, in the course of a few years, become part of life for all health professionals. The rapidity of this development has led to much confusion about the way audit should be conducted, and to concerns about the impact audit will have on the professional lives of health care staff. This book addresses these problems. It shows that audit is under the control of individual health care professionals and provides a powerful tool which can be used to modify practice in the ways which practitioners decide is best for their patients. The book reviews the methods which can be used, from simple case presentations to multi-centre data collection, and indicates how to select the one most suited to local circumstances.

This book provides a complete guide to the design and conduct of successful audit studies. It makes illustrative use of published audits from a range of specialties, from which detailed practical advice is developed. Each chapter has a short introduction to its contents and a summary of the key points at the end. Chapters 1 and 2 introduce audit and outline its simple underlying principles. Chapters 3 to 5 show how audit studies can be managed effectively; how important topics are identified; and how standards of care are set. Chapters 6 and 7 describe the methods of audit, reviewing the practical issues of collecting and processing accurate and useful data. Chapter 8 addresses the difficult area of bringing about change in the delivery of health care. It reviews methods for effecting change, describing how successful strategies for promoting change can be developed and implemented. Chapter 9 outlines the statistical techniques for data analysis, and points out the pitfalls for the interpretation of audit studies. Finally, Chapter 10 draws the previous chapters together in a step-by-step guide to the design of feasible and effective audit studies.

The book is intended for individuals or small groups from any of the health care professions who wish to undertake audit. The methods described are suitable for projects of any size, from the review of a few case notes to nationwide surveys. However, central to the approach of this book is the view that a small study which achieves a modest improvement in health care is to be preferred to a major data collection exercise. Large studies may describe many deficiencies in care, but remedy none. The book makes the essential distinction between measuring care and improving care. Audit begins by measuring care but its ultimate aim is to improve it.

Foreword

Medical or clinical audit is now an expected part of routine practice and the work of all clinicians. Its introduction was broadly welcomed but its implementation has caused some bewilderment and confusion. Concern for the care of individual patients has always been an objective of practitioners; the difference that audit brings is that it requires a systematic and critical analysis of valid measures of the quality of care so that changes can be made to improve care.

This new handbook of audit will be of value for everyone involved with the practicalities of medical and clinical audit. The authors have described with clarity the different stages of medical audit from the need for valid measures of quality, appropriate sample size and statistical rigour, to the need for simplicity and consideration of the behavioural aspects of implementing change. Written without resorting to 'quality speak', it provides clear definitions and descriptions of the technical terms associated with audit. The points made are illustrated with examples from the literature and from the authors' own experience. Practical points which should help audit groups are purposefully and usefully drawn together throughout the book. This is a book for clinicians concerned with improving their practice.

Clinical audit and quality assurance are the provenance of teams. The information contained in this book will have added value as it is shared. One of its major effects will be to promote discussion, debate and understanding about medical audit between members of clinical teams as audit becomes an integral part of the process of care.

This readable and comprehensive account is a *vade-mecum* of audit.

Fiona Moss
Editor, *Quality in Health Care* and Consultant Physician
Central Middlesex Hospital NHS Trust
London

Acknowledgements

Many of the ideas expressed in this book were developed during research and audit studies carried out with the North British Pain Association and funded by The Clinical Resource and Audit Group (CRAG) of The Scottish Office, and The Ian Mactaggart Trust. We are very grateful for their support and assistance. We thank our friends and colleagues for helpful suggestions and comments on this book, in particular Drs Fiona Williams and James Donnelly, and Mr Alistair Fogg. We also thank Catherine Grant for her patient proofing.

1

The Development of Audit

INTRODUCTION

Clinical audit is concerned with improving the quality of medical care. In this it is not new: codes of practice in medicine date back thousands of years and the most well known, the Hippocratic oath, was by no means the first. What is new is the scale of audit activities as a result of the 1989 Government White Paper *Working For Patients*, with its commandment *physician audit thyself*. An editorial in the British Medical Journal captured the prevailing mood: *'doctors in Britain have hummed and hawed over audit for years, but now everybody is supposed to be doing it'* [1]. A bewildering array of methods are being used and *'many doctors are far from clear about what exactly they should be doing'*.

The Working Paper which followed the White Paper was concerned mainly with the organisation of audit activities, clarifying where responsibilities lay for ensuring that audit was carried out and that remedial action was taken where necessary. The professions were, quite deliberately, left to decide the specific features of audit, such as the aspects of health care which should be audited and the methods which should be used. This neatly side-stepped the potential minefield of a government attempting to prescribe to doctors, and allowed the individual doctor to develop methods most appropriate to local circumstances. Unfortunately this tactic has created a new set of problems. There are many approaches to audit, and almost as many views on how audit should be conducted as there are authors on the subject. Care needs to be taken in the selection of topics and methods, to ensure that each study achieves what is intended. The ultimate aim of audit, that it should lead to improvements in patient care, is perhaps the only aspect on which there is consensus. The big—and as yet unanswered—question about all the current activity is whether it will lead to improved care, or whether it will be another illustration of a common failing: the confusion of activity with progress.

This chapter introduces clinical audit and the events which shaped it and led to the current widespread interest. It is not intended to provide a comprehensive review of the history of audit, because we are more interested in the present than the past. Instead it identifies several key developments in audit which introduce important concepts and the principal methods of audit. A colleague described audit as *'worthy but dull'*. We hope that this chapter will confirm that it is worthwhile and, if not always thrilling, it is sometimes exciting and always challenging and rewarding.

EARLY EXAMPLES OF AUDIT

The exploration begins with two examples of audit involving an English nurse in the mid-19th Century and an American surgeon in the early 20th Century. It is curious that concerns about the quality of medical care in a peninsula in the Black Sea and in the United States can illustrate so many facets of the purposes and methods of audit.

Debacle in the Crimea

The Crimean war began in 1854 when Britain and France invaded the peninsula on the north coast of the Black Sea to help Turkey in its struggle with Russia. After initial success at the Battle of Alma River, casualties began rising at the subsequent siege of the Russian naval base at Sebastopol. The mortality of soldiers in the nearby British hospitals was scandalous. At its worst in January 1855 there were 3168 deaths in hospital, 83 from wounds, 2761 from infectious disease and 324 from other causes [2]. A report in *The Times* described some of the problems: '*Not only are there not sufficient surgeons ... not only are there no dressers and nurses ... there is not even linen to make bandages*' [3]. This led to widespread popular and political concern, which intensified when it was revealed that wounded French soldiers were given very much better care. Questions were asked in Parliament, Commissions of Enquiry formed, and '*a vote of censure on the government ... was carried in an uproar by a majority of 157. The government fell*'. One of the most significant results of the furore was that the Secretary at War asked Florence Nightingale, a society lady with a devotion to nursing, to lead a team of nurses to the military hospitals at Scutari, near Constantinople.

The conditions Nightingale found at Scutari were wretched. The lavatories at one hospital, the Barrack, were flooded with sewage because the water supply had been shut off and they could not be flushed. The water supply to the greater part of the hospital was contaminated because it passed through the decaying carcass of a horse. In addition to fleas, rats and open sewers Nightingale found filthy linen, inedible food and a shortage of medical and surgical supplies. For example during a cholera epidemic she estimated that there were more than 1000 men suffering from acute diarrhoea but only 20 chamber pots. There was also a shortage of operating facilities: men were operated on in the wards on trestle tables in front of their waiting colleagues.

The problems were due to a chronic shortage of money allied to a cumbersome bureaucracy. Responsibility for the hospitals was unclearly divided among three agencies who, as the disaster unfolded, were more concerned to deny the existence of the problems and any responsibility for them than to remedy them. The problems were formidable, but Florence Nightingale was more than Longfellow's figure of the '*lady with a lamp*'. She was an indomitable, resourceful woman who wrought a revolution in the delivery of medical care at Scutari. Her response was to take direct action where she could, using her private income and money from a fund established by *The Times*. One of her first actions was to establish an extra kitchen in her own apartments to prepare food which could be digested by wounded soldiers. A different form of problem was the opposition she met from the doctors who were understaffed and overworked and thought it *'the last straw that a young Society lady should be foisted on them with a pack of nurses'* [3]. With one exception they made no use of the nurses. Nightingale's approach here was to win confidence gradually and let the doctors discover that she and her nurses could be of benefit to them. She also documented the appalling conditions in reports to influential friends including the Secretary at War and subsequently the Prime Minister. Gradually changes were made: the sanitation was improved, and Nightingale established a laundry and became quartermaster for the hospital to ensure adequate delivery of supplies. Her achievements show her considerable courage and determination but she also took full advantage of her social position to influence the authorities.

The example of Scutari is remarkable for two reasons. The first is the pioneering use of detailed reports on the quality of medical care to persuade politicians, generals and administrators of the need for change. This weapon was of enduring power, for Nightingale used it to good effect in military hospitals throughout Britain and India. Others also took it up: a disconcerting finding of one committee of enquiry was that the closer a regiment was based to the Barrack Hospital the higher the mortality it experienced. The second remarkable point is that, although it took heroic effort, changes actually took place in the delivery of health care. At its worst, over 40% of the soldiers admitted to hospital died there; within six months of Nightingale's arrival the death rate had fallen to 2%. To achieve this she used a mixture of guile, persuasion and political influence. It may appear strange that there could be resistance to change in the face of such appalling conditions, but there was and it was entrenched. Commonly, identifying deficiencies in care is very much easier than achieving their remedy.

The problems of the hospital at Scutari may appear too extreme and too remote to have much significance today, but nonetheless they illustrate some of the basic features of modern audit. Firstly, a health care problem is identified often by comparison with another area, in this case the treatment of the wounded French soldiers. The deficiencies in the delivery of care are carefully documented both to identify the required actions and to use the documented evidence to help bring about change. Implementing change was difficult and a variety of strategies were required. For the administrators the mixture was determination, guile and external support. For doctors the changes were planned and implemented with sensitivity, the guiding principle being that individuals who have to change their behaviour should believe that it is in their own interests to do so. These features and others essential to audit will be explored in more detail throughout this book.

Diploma mills and deplorable surgery

The late 19th Century was a time of rapid development of surgical techniques with the combination of anaesthetics and antisepsis leading to dramatic improvements in treatment. In the United States by the turn of the century there was concern that many doctors were poorly trained and *'were giving surgery a bad name because of their lack of skill'* [4]. Medical schools at this time were profit-making institutions and readily accepted poorly qualified students, who were then licensed to practice after two or three years teaching which included little clinical experience. The scale of the problem was exposed in 1910 in a report for the Carnegie Foundation by Abraham Flexner who, as Lembcke put it, *'did not mince words'* [4]. A quote from Flexner's report gives an indication of the trenchant comments made: *'a wretched hospital, really a death trap, heavily laden with debt, and without laboratory equipment enough to make an ordinary clinical examination'*.

Flexner's study, with its careful documentation of existing problems, led to major reforms. Medical education was moved from the *'diploma mills'* to universities, and given a proper scientific and clinical foundation. The survey also led to the establishment of an accrediting organisation for surgeons in 1913, the

American College of Surgeons, whose primary aim was to improve the standards of the profession. This early use of accreditation as a means of ensuring standards is a major landmark and is now a characteristic of the approach to quality of medical care in the United States.

Flexner's review of the quality of care in medical schools led to disquiet about the non-teaching hospitals. In 1916 the founder director of the American College of Surgeons, J G Bowman, carried out a second more extensive survey of all large hospitals. A significant development was the use of objective assessments of the quality of care delivered: for selected conditions, the elements of diagnosis and treatment which constitute good management were specified in advance of the study. The management of individual patients was then compared against these criteria. The use of objective criteria is one of the vital components of successful audit (see Chapter 5). Certainly Bowman's survey was successful in identifying deficiencies in the delivery of care: only 89 of 692 large hospitals were able to meet reasonable standards of care. Unfortunately the report was a victim of its own success: *'Although the College made the numbers public, it burned the list of hospitals at midnight in the furnace of the Waldorf Astoria Hotel, New York, to keep it from the press. Some of the most prestigious hospitals in the country had failed to meet the most basic standards'* [5]. The College of Surgeons had decided that publication would not be in the public interest.

The response of the College of Surgeons to the problems Bowman had unearthed was to define minimum standards for hospitals. To encourage hospitals to meet these standards, a list of approved or accredited hospitals was to be published. In the event the publication of the list was delayed by the hospitals who did not meet the standards, but this is a minor point. The main point is that a Hospital Standardisation Program had been established and it was an undoubted success in improving the quality of care offered by hospitals. With its success the Program expanded. Initially it was restricted to surgeons but in 1951 several other medical colleges joined the Program to form the Joint Commission on Accreditation of Hospitals [5]. The Program also expanded the scope and detail of the specifications, so that what began in 1919 with a single sheet of five points had become a 152 page manual by 1970. In 1966 the thrust of the standards was changed so that they specified an optimal achievable level rather than simply an essential minimum. Finally, the scope of coverage was extended to include not just hospitals but also community and ambulatory health care.

There is much to be learned from this American experience. First, the accreditation program gradually evolved from limited beginnings until, through negotiation, it embraced the whole profession. Thus whatever approaches are adopted, they should be tested on a limited scale and only if successful be applied more extensively. The present danger of the rush to audit is that poorly tested methods will be widely implemented, only to be found unable to deliver the expected return of improved patient care.

The second point concerns the value of defined standards of care. These allow us to identify with more certainty instances of inadequate care and clarify the standards which should be achieved.

A final, somewhat less direct, point is the need for confidentiality of the details of audit studies. We saw that the College of Surgeons decided not to publish Bowman's report. Although this could be criticised as a cynical political act, it may have been a better option than publication. There is an important distinction between the overall findings of a study and the details which might identify individuals or institutions. The surgeons published the findings, but more importantly acted to remedy the problems. Although it might be argued that those who offer inadequate care deserve to be identified, there are two important reasons why this is not the case. The first is the practical one that unless the results were to be kept confidential many clinicians, and perhaps especially those concerned about possible findings, would refuse to take part. The second is that the aim of audit, to improve patient care, is more likely to be hindered than helped by threats of public exposure and disciplinary action. Voluntary cooperation to achieve shared objectives is likely to be a more effective strategy; complete confidentiality is a cornerstone of modern audit.

A LESSON FROM AMERICA

The Americans have now had over 70 years' experience of audit, and have spent many hundreds of millions of dollars on it. The development of audit in the UK might thus follow the American model. This view is sometimes proposed in the UK, but as the next example illustrates there are several reasons why this might not be desirable.

One of the most significant of the bewildering array of developments in audit in the USA was the formation of Professional Standards Review Organisations (PSROs). As with many audit initiatives in the United States, PSROs have their origins in public and political concerns about an emerging crisis [6]. This time the problems lay with the Medicare and Medicaid programs which provide Federal funding for the health care of the poor and the elderly. By the late 1960s there was convincing evidence that many unnecessary investigations and treatments were being carried out. Further, the costs of these programs were spiralling, apparently out of control.

The problem was particularly acute in New York, where it has also been well documented [7]. One form of scam, which we should stress involved only a minority of doctors, was setting up so-called Shared Health Facilities (SHF). Typically an entrepreneur would rent and equip a suite of offices in one of the poorest parts of the city and recruit a multidisciplinary team, say a GP, a psychiatrist, a podiatrist, a gynaecologist, an optometrist and a chiropractor. Winsten has described the result: *'as a patient makes his way through a SHF, he is "ping-ponged" ... from practitioner to practitioner. Each provider examines the patient, subjects him to diagnostic tests, prescribes drugs, and urges him to return for a follow-up visit. Each practitioner bills Medicaid individually for the services provided, and returns a percentage of his earnings to the entrepreneur'* [7].

The existing mechanisms were clearly unable to prevent this and other types of over-utilisation, and legislation was passed in 1972 to create a nationwide network of Professional Standards Review Organisations (PSROs). Their initial remit covered both the costs and the quality of care delivered, but as the program developed the emphasis was increasingly given to costs. The program attempted to monitor the hospital stay of every Medicare and Medicaid patient and involved local practising physicians in the assessment of the appropriateness of the management. To enable these assessments to be carried out data were collected on investigations, treatments, complications and lengths of stay. Clearly the program was far from cheap; one estimate placed it at almost one billion dollars between 1972 and 1990 [8].

The PSRO program ran into a series of problems, with heated debate about its effects and effectiveness. The startling claim that it cost $1.80 for every $1 saved may have been disputed [6], but it illustrates the extent to which some commentators believe it had failed. From our point of view there are several features which do not commend it as a method of audit. The first is that the program was imposed by the government on the profession; the structure of the program was formalised at national level, with implementation being left to local initiatives. This led to considerable difficulties in the management of the program and to limited compliance. Secondly the program was rushed from design stage to implementation at a national level within two years. It is not surprising that the problems of implementation and of coping with the huge volumes of data were not fully appreciated. Even after several years of operation one of the early leaders of the program identified a number of problems including: lack of expertise among the program staff, poor data quality, inadequate methods for quality control and, not surprisingly, difficulties in changing physician behaviour [9].

Yet PSROs were not an unmitigated disaster. They still exist in the modified form of Peer Review Organisations, and are almost certainly effective at least as far as controlling costs. Nevertheless the precipitate development of large scale quality control programmes is unlikely to meet with immediate success.

Relevance of the American experience

The US health care services are quite different to those in Britain, precluding the direct transfer of their methods of audit. US medical records are of a high quality and can be used for audit much more readily than our own. High quality of case-notes has been a requirement of the accreditation program since its inception and, as the program expanded, medical records became increasingly important in the evaluation of quality of care. Medical records staff in the United States are more highly trained, are accorded a higher status and are much better paid than their British counterparts. It should be no surprise then that, although the Americans can use case-notes for audit, there are difficulties in doing so in Britain. In fact the quality of case-notes is a popular topic for audit in Britain, with the common finding that it is poor. Efforts are being made to remedy this but things still have a long way to go.

A second important contrast between the health services in Britain and the USA is in the method of funding. The American method is complex, involving a variety of agencies, and requires detailed information on the diagnosis and management of each patient. This is handled using computer systems which have grown in sophistication with the payment system. The cost of health care administration is far from small, consuming over 20% of all spending on health care [10]. Given that the data are already collected it is clearly sensible to use them for audit. Because the collection methods are in place it is possible, at little extra cost, to collect additional data more directly relevant to audit. In consequence much of the audit in the USA has involved large databases, often for tens of thousands of patients, using sophisticated computer systems to process the data. The danger of reviewing the American approach is that it might lead us to think that these large routine data collection systems are the best way to carry out audit. This is simply not true; Schumacher's thesis that small is beautiful applies with equal force in audit. The most cost-effective approach to audit is to collect limited data on a small but sufficient number of patients [11].

A final caveat on the American experience is that the thrust of the audit activity during the sixties and seventies was to control mushrooming costs rather than to improve patient care. A review by the Institute of Medicine of the National Academy of Sciences in 1990 concluded that even within the Medicare program: *'the current system to assess and ensure quality is in general not very effective and may have serious unintended consequences'* [12] .

Changing focus of audit in America

One aspect of the American experience from which we can learn is the way in which it developed. Although it is somewhat of a simplification, we can identify three phases in it. The first phase followed from Flexner's survey and focused on the provision of properly organised, trained staff with the necessary facilities to diagnose and treat patients. The implicit assumption was that, without these features, poor quality medical care would result. In the early days when there were serious deficiencies in the facilities provided, this assumption was undoubtedly true. Unfortunately today, although the lack of ideal facilities makes it more difficult to provide good medical care, the possession of them does not guarantee it. The quality and cost of the care delivered depends at least as much on the way facilities are used as on their quality.

The second phase of American audit focused on the way care was being delivered. Here the implicit assumption was that if care were adequate, the well-being of the patient was automatically guaranteed. This assumption has been increasingly challenged and has led to the third phase of audit which is primarily concerned with the outcome of patient care [13]. One result is that measures of outcome have been added to the standards set by the regulatory bodies [14]. Assessing outcome is far from simple and an initiative was launched in 1985 to develop measures of outcome. The research programme is spending vast sums of money in the process: $30 million in 1990 [13].

THE DEVELOPMENT OF AUDIT IN BRITAIN

Concern with quality of health care has been a feature of the National Health Service since its foundation in 1948. At this time the primary concern was with the evident deficiencies in the available facilities: *'in the beginning of the NHS planning for quality came to be mainly associated with the provision of "plant", i.e., buildings, equipment etc., and manpower provision, following comparisons with what was available elsewhere, either in the UK or abroad. The relative efficacy of this aspect of the service could be evaluated easily, especially since in the post-war period much of the "plant" tended to be outdated; and in certain places services did not exist'* [15]. Thus in the UK there were similar concerns to those in the USA some 30 years earlier. Undoubtedly the problems were not as severe as in the USA and also the motivation was different. In Britain the concern was to ensure that the whole population had access to the same high level of care, whereas in the USA the prime motivation was cost containment and, more recently, litigation avoidance.

An early audit in General Practice

One early study, which is more than a little reminiscent of the work of Flexner, was the survey of general practice by Collings in 1950 [16] which found much poor quality care. Collings wrote *'my observations have led me to write what is indeed a con-demnation of general practice in its present form'*. Collings was aware of the parallels to Flexner's work; he quoted a highly critical passage concluding: *'Flexner's description of medical practice in the last decades of the 19th century is almost a perfect word-picture of general practice as I found it in the industrial areas of England in 1949'*. The parallel continued because, as Flexner's study led to the formation of the American college of Surgeons, so Collings' survey gave impetus to the formation of the (now Royal) College of General Practitioners in 1952 [17].

Reducing maternal mortality

Collings's study, although it may have catalysed developments in general practice, did not itself lead directly to changes in the delivery of care. This is because the study simply observed current practice. Studies which are set up just to ask whether all is well, will in general not bring about change should all prove not to be well. An advance on this approach is seen in the Confidential Enquiry into Maternal Deaths [18] which focused on the reasons for inadequate care.

The origins of the enquiries into maternal mortality again lay in public anxiety about deaths, which led Neville Chamberlain to set up a Departmental Committee in 1929. Reports on maternal mortality were produced from 1932, but their quality was unreliable and they did not assess the quality of care for individual women. From 1952 standard data were collected, and although the system was voluntary it tried to cover all maternal deaths. The data were reviewed by independent experts at regional and national level to identify cases in which management was unsatisfactory. One early finding from the standardised data was of a high level of avoidable mortality among women with a retained placenta following a home delivery. Of 53 deaths associated with placental retention in the first three years of the enquiry, 89% had avoidable factors and many had been taken directly to hospital before adequate treatment (transfusion or removal of the placenta) had been given. Obstetric flying squads, which existed in some centres, were introduced to all regions with the policy of early treatment of these cases. As a result the number of such deaths in the next three year period fell from 53 to 24, and the proportion with avoidable factors fell from 89% to 48%.

These periodic enquiries into maternal mortality led to increasingly precise guidelines for patient management and helped to create a climate in which improvements in care could be implemented. It was decided at an early stage to publish the main findings of the enquiries (but not the individual details), despite concerns that there might be public criticism and a loss of confidence among pregnant women. In the event the reports were very well received by the health professions, and led to the establishment of similar studies in Northern Ireland, Scotland, New Zealand and Australia. Features of the enquiry which contributed to its success were:

● The scheme was voluntary. Compliance was enhanced because it was stressed that reports were treated with complete confidentiality and would not be used for disciplinary actions. It may be a reflection of the success of the scheme that these ideas have been embodied in most recent audit advice.

- A standard data collection form was used in all centres. Thus comparable data were obtained, and trends which could not be identified at a regional level because of small numbers became clear at the national level.
- The analysis was conducted at both regional and national levels. The main purpose of the enquiry was to encourage local review of the findings so that management changes, such as the increased awareness of toxaemia, could be introduced locally.

Recent developments in Britain

The Enquiry into Maternal Deaths was one of few early initiatives on the quality of health care. The history of audit in Britain is less one of continuous development as in the United States than of general indifference peppered by rare success. Undoubtedly concerns about the quality of care did develop but they did not have official sanction and audit was not widely practised. It was not until the publication of the *Cogwheel* report in 1967 that audit was recognised *'as a proper function for practising clinicians'* [19]. But even though an activity is proper, it may not be carried out. Concerns that Britain was not becoming involved in audit were still being expressed in the early seventies. The lack of effective mechanisms for ensuring quality of care was highlighted by a comment on *'the impotence of the General Medical Council, even in the face of flagrant abuse, was seen in its inability to constrain doctors who were over-prescribing heroin and other addictive drugs to their patients'* [20].

One feature of the development of audit in Britain is the changing role of government. In the late 1960s political involvement was direct, as for example in the UK national quality control scheme for clinical chemistry analyses in hospital laboratories [21]. A further example was the establishment of the Hospital Advisory Service (HAS) in 1969 [22]. The then Minister of Health, Richard Crossman, took a leading role, possibly because, as in previous examples, there was an emerging disaster. As Baker put it, the service was set up *'following a series of scandals and investigations in psychiatric hospitals.'* The method used is worth reviewing because it is the antithesis of the massive data collection approach of the Professional Standards Review Organisations (PSROs). Instead hospitals were visited by a multidisciplinary team of doctors, nurses and administrative staff who would inspect all parts of the hospital and talk to as many of the staff as possible. Problems identified and possible solutions were discussed at the end of the visit by the visiting team and the hospital staff. The experience of the HAS is that the most fruitful discussions were those which involved all the staff rather than those dominated by a few. Acknowledging the existence of problems in a multidisciplinary environment is an important first step towards resolving them. Baker commented: *'a multidisciplinary team of administrator, medical, nursing, remedial and social work staff was more likely to commit all the professions involved to any real change or progress, and having once committed themselves to this system, found there were significant benefits'* [22].

Since then Government involvement has been less direct although Royal Commissions in 1976 (the Alment report) and 1979 (the Merrison report) emphasised the importance of audit. Instead it was the Royal Colleges themselves who took the active role. In 1975 the Radiologists established a working party on the use of diagnostic radiology [23], and in 1977 the Physicians founded the Medical Services Group essentially to carry out audit [24]. A chronological summary of these and other developments, most notably in Nursing and in General Practice, is given in Table 1.1. It is beyond the scope of this chapter to review all of these in detail. The important point is that there was considerable interest and activity in audit many years before the 1989 White Paper.

The introduction of audit was slow, however, being delayed in part by professional inertia but also by some active resistance [25–27]. One understandable concern was with the possible loss of clinical freedom. However, a cardinal feature of good clinical audit is that it is completely under the control of the healthcare professional, who uses it as a tool to advise on whether changes in practice are required.

During the last decade the audit movement has gathered speed, with an increasing number of individual enthusiasts becoming involved, in addition to the professional bodies discussed above.

Table 1.1 *Some important developments affecting the quality of medical care in Britain*

Year	Organisation	Activity
1952	Royal College of Obstetricians and Gynaecologists	*Confidential Enquiry into Maternal Deaths* put on sound footing
1952	College of General Practitioners founded	One founding aim was to improve patient care
1967	Ministry of Health	*Cogwheel* report established audit as a proper function for doctors
1969	The Hospital Advisory Service established	Led to improved patient management in psychiatric hospitals
1969	United Kingdom national quality control scheme	Monitored the quality of clinical chemistry analyses in hospital laboratories
1975	Royal College of Radiologists	Established working party on use of diagnostic radiology
1976	Committee of Enquiry Report *Competence to Practice* (Alment Report)	Stated that doctors should review their work regularly with their colleagues
1977	Royal College of Physicians founded the Medical Services Group	Carried out studies intended to lead to improvements in medical care
1978	Conference of Senior Hospital Staff	Passed resolution on medical audit
1978	Royal College of Nursing	Established working party on standards of care
1979	Royal Commission on National Health Service (Merrison Report)	Emphasised the importance of audit
1980	Royal College of General Practitioners	Took initiative on quality of service in general practice
1984	WHO health policy	Government signs declaration that effective mechanisms for quality of health care will be in place by 1990
1985	Royal College of General Practitioners	Issued policy statement *Quality in General Practice*
1987	Royal College of Surgeons	Requirement that regular audit was necessary for training posts to be recognised
1989	Royal College of Physicians	Report on Medical Audit
1989	Department of Health	White Paper *Working for Patients*

THE NEED FOR AUDIT

The institutional and individual developments in audit culminated in the publication of the White Paper *Working For Patients* in 1989, which stated that all doctors should become involved in audit. A subsequent NHS circular in 1990 extended the coverage to nursing, and the other health care professions have followed. The resistance to audit which was voiced in the early seventies has mostly been replaced by growing enthusiasm. Audit has now become orthodox and many of the Royal Colleges stipulate that training posts for junior staff will only be recognised if there is an active audit programme within the unit. Although many health care professionals may regard these as dramatic developments, they are no more than the natural progression of a movement which has been gathering momentum over the last 20 years.

Although there is official encouragement for all doctors and other health professionals to audit their practice it would be unfortunate only to do so out of necessity. There are several cogent arguments which underline the value of audit. More importantly, it is only when the need for audit has been identified that it becomes clear what should be done; the approach and the methods follow directly from the purposes. There are several distinct arguments to consider.

Variation in the care delivered

The wide geographical differences in the delivery of health care form a compelling reason for audit. The nub of the problem is contained in the title of a paper by Wennberg and colleagues [28]: *'Are hospital services rationed in New Haven or over-utilised in Boston ?'*. This problem is not restricted to the USA. For example Wilkin and Smith [29] reported that the frequency with which general practitioners referred patients to hospital ranged from less than one per hundred consultations to over sixteen per hundred; McPherson and colleagues found a two-fold variation in the rates of some surgical operations [30]; and Fowkes and McPake found over a three-fold variation between the regions in England and Wales in attendances at out-patients [31]. As is clear from the title of Wennberg's paper, we cannot say what is the appropriate level of medical activity, but it is certain that not all are correct.

Limitation of resources

A cornerstone of health economics is that resources are limited, so that the best possible use of resources must be made to meet the demand for health care. This does not just apply to those planning health care who have to balance the competing claims of, for example, coronary artery by-pass surgery and kidney dialysis. It also applies to the individual doctor when deciding how to allocate time between patients and which investigative procedures and management strategies to choose. A good example of the way in which audit can be used to identify unnecessary procedures comes from the initiative taken by the Royal College of Radiologists [32]. They conducted a survey of the use of pre-operative chest X-rays (POCR) in over 10000 patients undergoing non-acute, non-cardiopulmonary surgery. The study involved eight hospitals throughout Britain, and found that the frequency of POCR varied markedly between hospitals (11.5% to 54.2%) and could not be explained by differences in the types of operation. Of more concern was that the results of radiography had no apparent influence on the decision to operate nor on the choice of anaesthetic. The immediate conclusions about the frequency of unnecessary radiography led to the development of guidelines by the College, and to the recommendation that the frequency of use of POCR need not be higher than the lowest observed in the study (11.5%).

Evident deficiencies in the care delivered

Human fallibility has long been recognised but few have systematically studied their errors as Sir Humphry Davy commended in the early 19th Century: *'I thank God I was not made a dextrous manipulator; the most important of my discoveries have been suggested to me by my failures'* [33]. The most direct evidence of the need for audit comes from studies which have identified deficiencies in care which have subsequently been remedied. There are numerous examples of these which will be discussed in detail throughout this book, but it is worth outlining the approach with two examples. A survey of children in hospital being fed by intravenous catheter showed that in 45% of the cases the catheter had to be removed because of sepsis [34]. Management protocols were modified and the staff were given intensive training. A subsequent period of monitoring gave the gratifying result that now only 8% of catheters were becoming infected. A similar approach to the treatment of major trauma patients led to the frequency of management errors falling from 58% to 30% [35].

Organisational need for audit

Any large organisation needs to monitor the quality of the work it does. Industry spends large sums on quality control because they are repaid by higher efficiency and hence greater profits. After its decimation in the Second World War, Japanese industry invested heavily in quality control, adopting what is now called Total Quality Management (TQM). This concern with quality contributed in large part to the well known resurgence of that country's economy. TQM involves much more than just inspection of the quality of components on a production line [36]. It represents a philosophy of approach which deals with individuals, providing them with the training and support to improve quality.

Technological advance and medical education

One of the subsidiary aims of audit is education. Medical science is advancing rapidly, making it difficult for professionals to keep up to date and increasing the likelihood that some will not. It should be clear from the examples in this chapter that audit can supply not only the means to identify such problems, but also a method to convey new information.

Political power of audit data

Several of the examples in this chapter have demonstrated the power of documented evidence of deficiencies in care to bring about major changes. A convincing argument for additional resources is evidence of deficiencies in care which could be remedied by those resources. Audit can provide data on unmet needs or lack of facilities, which may prove a stout defence against unevaluated changes proposed by management.

SUMMARY

This review has charted the key developments which have shaped audit. Several lessons can be learnt from this history in the United States and Britain:

- Audit is not just another administrative nuisance imposed by interfering politicians; it has been employed effectively for many years.
- There is strong evidence of deficiencies in health care which need to be rectified. There may be many more of which we are unaware.
- Monitoring the details of all patients is vastly expensive and has only a limited effect on the quality of patient care.
- The major problem is not identifying inadequate care, but changing clinical practice to improve patient care.
- Systems of audit which are developed rapidly with widespread implementation may be ineffective. The speed with which audit has been introduced in Britain increases the likelihood that some audit activities may be ineffective. There may be a lot of audit about, but that does not mean that all of it is good.
- Audit is sometimes viewed as threatening, but it should be under the complete control of the individual clinician, who can use it as a powerful tool to assist in providing care to the highest standards.
- Audit can be effective if carried out at a local level with the cooperation and support of all relevant professional groups.

The rest of this book develops the knowledge and skills which will enable health care professionals to carry out successful audit.

REFERENCES

1. Moss F, Smith R. From audit to quality and beyond. Br Med J 1991; 303: 199–200.
2. Cohen IB. Florence Nightingale. Sci Am 1984; 250: 98–107.
3. Smith CW. Florence Nightingale. London: Constable, 1950.
4. Lembcke PA. Evolution of the Medical Audit. J Am Med Assoc 1967; 199: 111–18.
5. Roberts JS, Coale JG, Redman RR. A history of the Joint Commission on the Accreditation of Hospitals. J Am Med Assoc 1987; 258: 936–40.
6. Smitts HL. The PSRO in perspective. N Engl J Med 1981; 305: 253–9.
7. Winsten JA. Regulating shared health facilities in New York city. In: Greene R, ed. Assuring quality in medical care. Cambridge, Massachusetts: Ballinger, 1976: 195–211.
8. Anonymous. Legislated clinical medicine. Lancet 1990; 335: 1004–6.
9. Jonas S, Rosenberg SN. Measurement and control in the quality of health care. In: Jonas S, ed. Health care delivery in the United States. New York: Springer, 1986: 416–64.
10. Schroeder SA. Outcome assessment 70 years late: are we ready? N Engl J Med 1987; 316: 160–1.
11. Crombie IK, Davies HTO. Audit in outpatients: entering the loop. Br Med J 1991; 302: 1437–9.
12. Lohr KN, Schroeder SA. A strategy for quality assurance in Medicare. N Engl J Med 1990; 322: 707–12.
13. Epstein AM. The outcomes movement—will it get us where we want to go? N Engl J Med 1990; 323: 266–9.
14. O'Leary DS. The Joint Commission looks to the future. J Am Med Assoc 1987; 258: 951–2.
15. McLachlan G. Introduction and perspectives. In: McLachlan G, ed. A Question of Quality. London: Oxford University Press, 1976: 3–20.
16. Collings JS. General Practice in England Today: A Reconnaissance. Lancet 1950; i: 555–85.
17. Hunt JH. The foundation of a college. J R Coll Gen Pract 1973; 23: 5–20.

18. Godber G. The confidential enquiry into maternal deaths. In: McLachlan G, ed. A Question of Quality. London: Oxford University Press, 1976: 24–33.

19. Williamson JD. Quality control, medical audit and the general practitioner. J R Coll Gen Pract 1973; 23: 697–706.

20. Dollery CT. The quality of health care. In: McLachlan G, ed. Challenges For Change. London: Oxford University Press, 1971: 3–32.

21. Whitehead T. Surveying the performance of pathological laboratories. In: McLachlan G, ed. A Question of Quality. London: Oxford University Press, 1976: 97–117.

22. Baker A. The Hospital Advisory Service. In: McLachlan G, ed. A Question of Quality. London: Oxford University Press, 1976: 203–216.

23. Roberts CJ. Annotation: towards the more effective use of diagnostic radiology: a review of the work of the Royal College of Radiologists' working party on the more effective use of diagnostic radiology, 1976 to 1988. Clin Radiol 1988; 39: 3–6.

24. Clarke C, Whitehead AGW. The contribution of the Medical Services Group of the Royal College of Physicians to improvement in care. In: McLachlan G, ed. Reviewing practice in medical care: steps to quality assurance. London: Nuffield Provincial Hospital Trust, 1981: 33–40.

25. Mourin K. Audit in general practice. J R Coll Gen Pract 1975; 25: 682–3.

26. Hall H. Say "no" to audit. World Medicine 1979; 14 (September 8): 21–2.

27. McNicol GP. A rather sad document. Br Med J 1979; 2: 844–8.

28. Wennberg JE, Freeman JL, Culp WJ. Are hospital services rationed in New Haven or over-utilised in Boston? Lancet 1987; i: 1185–8.

29. Wilkin D, Smith AG. Variation in general practitioners' referral rates to consultants. J R Coll Gen Pract 1987; 37: 350–3.

30. McPherson K, Strong PM, Epstein A, Jones L. Regional variations in the use of common surgical procedures: within and between England and Wales, Canada, and the United States of America. Soc Sci Med 1981; 15A: 273–88.

31. Fowkes FGR, McPake BI. Regional variations in outpatient activity in England and Wales. Comm Med 1986; 8: 286–91.

32. National Study by The Royal College of Radiologists. Preoperative chest radiology. Lancet 1979; ii: 83–6.

33. Strauss MB. Familiar Medical Quotations. Boston: Little, Brown, 1968.

34. Puntis JWL, Holden CE, Smallman S, Finkel Y, George RH, Booth IW. Staff training: a key factor in reducing intravascular catheter sepsis. Arch Dis Child 1990; 65: 335–7.

35. Fisher RB, Dearden CH. Improving the care of patients with major trauma in the accident and emergency department. Br Med J 1990; 300: 1560–3.

36. Neave HR. Deming's 14 points for management. The Statistician 1987; 36: 561–70.

2
Overview of Audit

INTRODUCTION

The literature on audit is vast and disparate in the methods used. The speed of development has led to much confusion, but there is one certain foundation on which an overview of audit can be built: the principal aim is to improve the quality of medical care. This is the one feature of audit for which there is agreement in review articles [1–4] and among the Royal Colleges [5–7]. However we need more than just the aim: a good definition should *describe a thing by its properties* [8]. Although none of the existing definitions covers the full range of properties of audit, it is useful to consider them to identify the true nature of audit. This chapter reviews these definitions, then provides an overview of audit, concluding with a summary of its essential characteristics.

The conventional definition

The definition of audit presented in the 1989 White Paper and now much repeated is singularly unhelpful: *'the systematic critical analysis of the quality of medical care, including the procedures used for diagnosis and treatment, the use of resources and the resulting outcome and quality of life for the patient'* This definition focuses on the areas to be assessed. It does not identify the purposes of audit nor suggest how studies are carried out. What it does identify is that audit involves a criticism of current practice and that the care given, the resources used, and the resulting benefit to the patient should all be assessed. This is an important point because it stresses that audit is intended to cover all aspects of health care. It is not restricted to the accuracy of diagnosis or the appropriateness of treatments given, but includes such diverse topics as the quality of referral letters, the timeliness of diagnostic tests, and the information given to patients about their disease.

The most troublesome word in this definition is *systematic*. Allied to the breadth of care which is to be assessed, the word systematic is sometimes taken to mean that assessment of care should be continuous and that all aspects of care should be monitored. This view is misplaced. To paraphrase, you can audit a few topics all of the time or many topics for a short time but you cannot audit everything all of the time. The trouble with continuous assessment is that it leads naturally to the establishment of routine data collection systems. Experience from the United States (see Chapter 1) is that such systems are extremely costly and often do not meet expectations.

Definition by method

Some authors have focused their definitions on the methods used to carry out audit. For example Slee [9], in the United States proposed: *'the evaluation of the quality of medical care as reflected in medical records'*. Ellis gives an alternative view when he describes audit as a computerised data processing system [10]. The limitation of these methodological definitions is that they fail to recognise that a variety of methods can be used in audit, each appropriate to local circumstances and the particular topic being investigated. These methods include case presentation, case-note review, *ad hoc* studies, criterion based audit, and occurrence screening (see Chapter 6).

Definitions of purpose

Purpose is a key element of many definitions of audit. For example Heath proposed *'the setting and maintenance of the highest possible standards appropriate for the situation'* [11]. A development of this, which indicates in part the method to be used, is the definition of Shaw and Costain: *'a systematic approach to peer review of medical care in order to identify opportunities for improvement and provide a mechanism for realising them'* [2]. Dixon [12] has taken this one stage further to define audit as: *'the systematic peer evaluation of the quality of patient care, based on explicit and measurable indicators of quality, for the purpose of demonstrating and improving the quality of patient care'*. This definition is more comprehensive, introducing the idea of measurement as well as purpose and method, but it is also somewhat of a mouthful. Yet even this is not all embracing; for example it gives no indication of what aspects of medical care should be audited nor how improvements in care can be implemented.

The supremacy of purpose

The foregoing definitions identify three distinct elements of audit: purpose, method, and area of investigation. Definitions which attempt to specify all three would be not only too long, they would also be unnecessarily restrictive: audit should cover all areas and use the most appropriate method for the subject in hand. Rather than attempt an all embracing and, in all probability, unreadable definition, we shall use one which identifies the primary purpose of audit: *audit is the process of reviewing the delivery of health care to identify deficiencies so that they may be remedied*. The rest of this chapter expands on the principles and characteristics of audit.

THE AUDIT CYCLE

Our definition of audit specifies the two key activities, the identification of the problem and the remedy for it, but leaves unanswered how deficiencies in health care are identified. The answer is by comparison of current practice against agreed standards. The use of standards of care in this way is characteristic of audit. These ideas are embodied in the audit cycle, shown in Figure 2.1, developed from Fowkes [13]. The natural starting point is the assessment of the quality of current care. Deficiencies in care can then be identified by comparing the care which is actually being delivered against the standard which has been set. Standards, then, are central to the conduct of audit and it is worth exploring them in a little detail here.

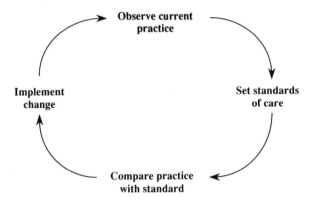

Figure 2.1   *The audit cycle*

The value of standards

An example of an audit of wound infection in major colorectal and biliary surgery illustrates the nature and uses of standards. Colorectal surgery is known to carry a significant risk of infection, but when one centre reviewed a series of cases it was surprised that the infection rate was as high as 43% [14]. Changes in the use of prophylactic antibiotics were introduced with a resulting fall in the rate to 18%. However when compared against a published series in which only a 7% infection rate was reported [15], it was clear that further improvements could be made.

In this example two types of standards were used. When the initial high infection rate was discovered, clinical experience was sufficient to indicate that there were deficiencies in care. Clinical judgement is being used as an unspoken or implicit standard, and can be sufficient when deficiencies are so large as to be self-evident. However as the level of care is improved it becomes more difficult to know whether what is being achieved is acceptable. This is when an explicit standard is useful; the reported value of 7% infected wounds gives a target at which to aim. Setting an explicit target has a second use; it ensures that the audit findings are not used merely to validate current practice (see Chapter 5). Setting standards is recognised to be an important but difficult stage of audit [16, 17] and is reviewed in detail in Chapter 5.

The importance of effecting change

The final step of the cycle, and the one which gives the rationale for audit, is to implement changes to improve the delivery of health care. There is no point in describing a health care problem if nothing is done to ameliorate it. However the first attempt at change is often only partially successful in resolving the problem: the example of wound infection showed an initial reduction in the wound infection rate from 43% to 20%, but, with additional improvements in antibiotic prophylaxis, the rate was eventually reduced to 2% [14]. This is why the steps in audit are displayed in Figure 2.1 as a cycle: to achieve the desired level of care it may be necessary to re-enter the cycle and repeat the steps. Unfortunately it is generally much easier to identify problems than to remedy them. There are many and subtle barriers to effecting change which, together with strategies to overcome them, are described in detail in Chapter 8.

OTHER CHARACTERISTICS OF AUDIT

The essential features of audit are embodied in the audit cycle but there are many other characteristics common to good audit. These are described in the following sections.

Education

The educational value of audit is recognised in many review papers [13, 18] but most particularly in the report of the Standing Committee on Postgraduate Medical Education [19]. The process of audit focuses attention on a particular feature of care, encouraging doctors to think critically about their practice and to discuss this with colleagues. More importantly it can provide the motivation to further education by highlighting areas of need. Since these issues are consequences of audit findings, rather than substantive issues which affect the design and conduct of audit studies, they will not be pursued further.

Confidentiality

A cornerstone of audit is that complete confidentiality is assured for the patients whose care is reviewed and the doctors who managed them. This was recognised in the 1989 White Paper which emphasised that audit should be led by doctors and that confidentiality of those involved should be ensured. Subsequent official papers dealing with nursing and the para-medical professions have reinforced this view. Audit will only be of value when the doctors involved are confident that the findings cannot be used for disciplinary proceedings.

The seriousness with which confidentiality is taken was demonstrated in a recent nationwide audit, the Confidential Enquiry into Peri-operative Death [20], which ensured that all assessments were conducted without the patient, doctor or institution being identified. *'Crown privilege'* was also obtained, such that it was deemed *'in the public interest'* that the data could not be subpoenaed by a court. Finally, just to make sure, all the original data were shredded before the findings of the study were released. Few audit studies will need to go to these lengths to ensure confidentiality, but the matter should be taken into account in the design of any study.

Multidisciplinary

Medical care is delivered jointly by several professions, so it follows that the audit of this care should involve the same groups. If one group conducts an audit in isolation, it may be difficult to implement the findings across professional boundaries. Instead, all of those who are involved in the care being audited should be part of the audit group from the beginning. An audit of central venous catheterisation for parenteral nutrition of children illustrates the advantages of multidisciplinary audit. Concern arose following a survey which found that 45% of catheters had to be removed because of sepsis [21]. Management of these patients involves many specialties including surgical and medical staff, nutritional and nursing teams, and microbiologists. All were involved in the development of management guidelines and of an educational programme, which was repeated regularly because of the high turn-over of medical and nursing staff. In the follow-up period after these initiatives the sepsis rate had fallen to 8%. Organising and managing audit studies is a much wider task than collecting data and drawing up guidelines. The design of the audit study needs to be discussed and the programme of action negotiated with all staff. Approaches for achieving this are fully reviewed in Chapter 3.

Relationship to management

Although audit is led by health professionals, local management has been set the responsibility of ensuring that *'an effective system of medical audit is in place'* [22]. By April 1991 a medical audit committee, chaired by a senior clinician, had to be established in each health district to *'plan and monitor a comprehensive plan of medical audit.'* The committee has to: agree its annual forward programme with the district general manager; ensure that deficiencies in care, when identified through audit, are remedied; and initiate independent audit where necessary.

The role of management is to facilitate the conduct of audit by recognising it as a legitimate activity for doctors. This includes providing resources for audit. Many district health authorities have appointed audit support staff, variously called audit assistants, officers, coordinators or facilitators [23]. In addition funds to support audit activities including the purchase of computers and associated software are usually available. Appropriately handled management can be a boon to audit; in principle they should never be an impediment or a hazard.

Service efficiency

In some instances reviewing health care can increase the efficiency of its delivery. When this occurs it is a bonus, however efficiency is not a primary aim of audit. Efficiency of health care is an arena in which doctors will increasingly be involved but it is separate from audit. It falls more readily under the heading Resource Management, and is a task conducted jointly with management. This is in contrast to audit whose conduct is under the complete control of health professionals, and whose aim is the provision of better care.

Designing effective audit

Audit is difficult and time-consuming so most individuals or groups will only be able to undertake a few studies each year. The range of potential studies is vast, and the problem is not of finding topics, but of selecting the most valuable ones for audit. In this way audit is like health care itself; the resources available are limited and decisions, sometimes difficult, have to be taken on which options to pursue. The temptation to get started quickly can lead to the collection of data without a clear purpose, so that much time and effort will be consumed to limited effect. Instead care should be taken to select an important topic and data collection should be focused on it. The rationale for selecting a topic follows from the definition of audit: the problem audited should be capable of change and if successful the change achieved should be worthwhile. There is clearly a subjective element to 'worthwhile' but a rough assessment can be made. Even a small audit project may involve 50 or 100 patients and take several months to complete. Larger studies can involve hundreds of patients and take years. The likely outcome can be viewed in terms of how many patients may benefit as a result of a successful audit. If a few patients will benefit greatly or many patients will benefit to some extent, then the audit may be justified. A more detailed review of criteria for selecting a topic is given in Chapter 4, and Chapter 6 outlines the approach for deciding how big a study should be. The stages in the design of effective audit studies are reviewed in Chapter 10.

One result from an audit study may be the identification of a health care problem which cannot be remedied immediately. This can happen when the remedy would involve considerable expenditure or when professionals in other disciplines are involved. This does not mean that the audit was a waste of time; the findings can be used as a powerful argument for additional resources: *'you cannot take sides against arithmetic'* (Winston Churchill)[24].

THE STAGES OF AN AUDIT STUDY

The audit cycle in Figure 2.1 describes the general approach to audit but does not identify the tasks which constitute audit. The cycle has been recast in Figure 2.2 to specify the activities to be carried out. At first sight this appears straightforward;

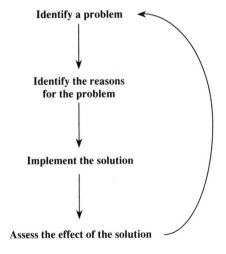

Figure 2.2   *The steps in an audit cycle*

the problem is identified, described in some detail and a solution implemented. However the apparent simplicity of this flowchart conceals an abundance of problems that arise in many audit studies. Clinical skills are essential when dealing with many of these problems, and much satisfaction can be had from solving them.

Confirm the problem

Audit often begins with a suspicion of a deficiency in health care which needs to be confirmed and, if possible, refined. An audit of death of children with head injuries illustrates the steps involved [25]. Head injury is a major cause of death in children and specialist neurosurgical centres reported fatality rates ranging from 6% to 35%. Although the range could in part reflect differences in the severity of patients seen, one group claimed that the fatality rate should not exceed 10%. Concern about this topic led to a survey of the management of fatal cases in the Northern region of England, which revealed that 32% of those dying in hospital had potentially avoidable factors which contributed to death. Among those who died before admission to hospital 22% had avoidable factors. The authors had confirmed that in many cases care was inadequate, but they were also able to identify where the deficiencies lay: in the delayed diagnosis of intracranial haemorrhage; inadequate management of airways; and inadequate management of transfer between hospitals.

The steps in confirming the existence of a health care problem are summarised in Figure 2.3. Suspicion of a possible problem originates from a combination of clinical experience and published reports. Alternatively problems may be identified from an analysis of data which have been collected on the patients being seen. Confirmation that the problem is real and warrants action may mean collecting more data to estimate its scale. Desirable standards of care need to be set as a benchmark against which the actual care provided can be compared. Methods of setting standards are discussed in Chapter 5, but in brief they involve a review of the literature and discussion among local clinicians.

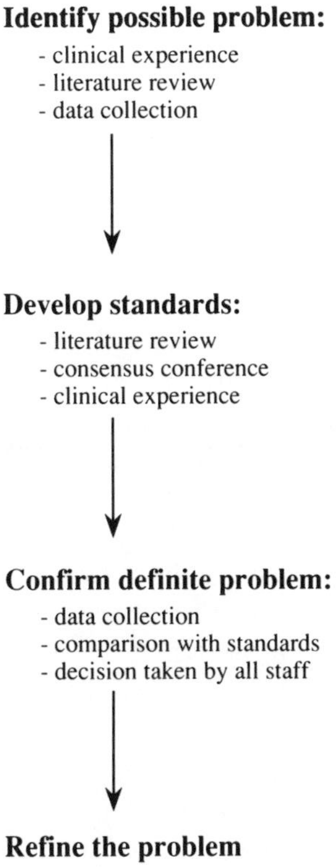

Identify possible problem:
- clinical experience
- literature review
- data collection

↓

Develop standards:
- literature review
- consensus conference
- clinical experience

↓

Confirm definite problem:
- data collection
- comparison with standards
- decision taken by all staff

↓

Refine the problem

Figure 2.3 *Confirming the existence of a health care problem*

One consequence of this process is that the nature of the problem is often considerably refined; for example Sharples and colleagues identified the specific management techniques which were unsatisfactory [25]. The refinement of the problem highlights the particular areas of care in which change needs to be effected. Successful audits have often adopted this careful reflective approach.

Identify the reasons for the problem

Confirming the existence of deficiencies in health care is quite different to knowing why they occurred. The study by Sharples and colleagues confirmed and refined the problem, but provided no illumination of the underlying cause. The obvious questions, why was diagnosis delayed and why was management inadequate, were not answered. As a consequence, their recommendation, that regional guidelines for optimal management of children with severe head injury should be revised, is general and a little vague. This may not be sufficient to remedy the problem; many studies have shown that the issuing of guidelines by themselves is often insufficient to influence clinician behaviour [26, 27].

A better approach was adopted in a study of the care of patients with major trauma in an accident and emergency department [28]. The study confirmed that management errors had occurred, and refined the nature of the problem: inappropriate treatment was more common in cases of blunt rather than penetrating trauma. However they also discovered the reasons: *'most errors occurred because these patients arrived outside ordinary office hours, when only inexperienced junior doctors staffed the department...[who] often failed to recognise the severity of the patients' injuries and consequently did not call for help from senior staff'.*

Identifying the root causes of the problem may involve additional data collection. This can include information on the nature of care given, the staff involved, the time and place of treatment, and the resources available. The types of questions that need to be asked are reviewed in detail in Chapter 8. The important point is that audit is an evolving process and the findings at one stage can determine what needs to be done at another. Audit studies need to be reassessed and modified in the light of preliminary findings.

Implement the solution

The changes which need to be effected in the delivery of care follow directly from the root causes of the deficiencies. For the study of major trauma, a severity score was developed to assist identification of severe injuries, and junior staff were encouraged to call out more senior colleagues to supervise the management of severe injuries. This solution was implemented, reducing the frequency of management errors by half.

Identifying the underlying causes of the deficiencies in care not only suggests the remedy, but enables it to be tailored exactly to the problem; in the major trauma study the management guidelines which were developed could highlight blunt trauma and be directed primarily towards junior doctors. General guidelines, which dealt with the whole area of major trauma, would not give emphasis to the problem area. The consequences of this study contrast with the earlier example of head injuries in children. In that study the root causes were not identified and a general solution was proposed but not implemented.

Assess the impact of the solution

Since audit is intended to improve patient care, the impact of proposed solutions needs to be assessed. This is usually referred to as closing the loop, and hence the process is termed the audit cycle. Obviously the methods by which the original problem was confirmed can be used to determine the change, but there is a difference. The most likely outcome of even a well conducted audit study is partial success. For example the audit of patients with major trauma could only reduce the frequency of management errors by half. In the audit of wound infection following colorectal surgery described above, two passes around the audit cycle were required to achieve an acceptable level of care. The scale of the remaining problem identified in the reassessment will indicate whether a further solution needs to be developed.

Therefore the assessment of the outcome of an audit should not just monitor the resulting quality of care, but should also try to determine why only partial success was achieved. There may be additional problems which were not evident during the first cycle of audit. Alternatively partial success could result from an inadequate implementation of the proposed solution. The extent of resistance to change by individuals and institutions is often not recognised in audit studies.

The full audit cycle

The steps in the full audit cycle are combined in Figure 2.4. The cycle may appear complex because of the cycle within a

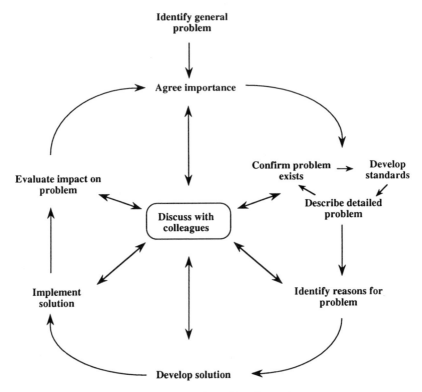

Figure 2.4   *The full audit cycle*

cycle, but this inner cycle is a crucial phase of successful audit. As a topic is studied the definition of the topic is refined and the standards of care which should be met are modified. In the process the standards to be met could also be refined. The inner cycle provides a key to successful audit: the identification of the underlying causes of the health care problem [29].

One of the principles of good audit is that regular discussions should be held with relevant staff as the project proceeds. Chapters 3 and 8 review in detail the needs and benefits of continual involvement of all staff in the audit project. Briefly, colleagues should be consulted or informed of developments at every stage, and be actively involved at certain key stages. The first of these is the assessment of the seriousness of the problem. If staff do not agree that the problem is an important one they are unlikely to develop and implement solutions.

Second, the standards against which the health care will be assessed need to be agreed. Otherwise if the standards are not met they may simply be discarded on the grounds that they were inappropriate. All staff should also be involved in the development of the solution. In general people are much more willing to co-operate in a venture for which they are responsible than one which is imposed from outside.

WHAT AUDIT IS NOT

The audit cycle described above not only clarifies the nature of audit, it also identifies those activities which are sometimes, in our view, incorrectly described as audit. It is not that these other activities are of no value, but confusing them with audit dissipates energies which could have been spent improving patient care.

Clinical research

Some authors [30] have suggested that audit is research and others have stated that it is not [12]. In part the disagreement arises because audit studies take advantage of many research techniques such as survey sampling, questionnaire design and statistical analysis. Both audit and research require well designed studies and both are concerned that sources of errors and bias do not compromise the findings.

Part of the confusion may occur because audit involves enquiry into the way health care is delivered, and enquiry could be seen as a synonym for research. However the motivations behind audit and research are quite different. Both involve the collection of data, but for audit the findings are often relevant only to local circumstances. Audit determines whether existing clinical knowledge, skills and resources are being properly used. In contrast, research is concerned with generating new knowledge which will have general application, as for example in determining whether a new treatment is superior to an existing one. The difference is between adding to the body of medical knowledge and ensuring that knowledge is effectively used. Audit is intended to influence the activities of an individual or a small team; clinical research seeks to influence medical practice as a whole.

A different way to look at this problem is to review what are termed the three Es of health care delivery: Efficacy, Effectiveness, and Efficiency. Efficacy involves assessing whether a treatment actually works and is the province of clinical research. Effectiveness is whether treatments which have been shown to work do so in practice; audit identifies instances where this does not happen so the problems may be rectified. Efficiency is whether resources are being used to best advantage and uses the techniques of health economics.

A survey

Many studies published as audit are little more than surveys of current practice. The findings are often interesting but, because an intention to effect change was not built into the study, few such studies lead directly to improvements in care.

A common defence of surveys is that they identify topics for audit. But most health professionals have a shrewd idea what is going on and will often not need a survey to find out where things are going wrong. Instead critical reflection on current practice and discussions with colleagues will identify many potential topics for audit. Approaches to generating and selecting topics are reviewed in Chapter 4.

Although audit is not a survey, surveys are indispensable for audit. This may seem paradoxical but the distinction lies in the purposes of the activity. Surveys provide the information needed for audit, which is then used to bring about change. Earlier examples showed that surveys can help quantify the size of the problem, refine its nature and help elucidate the underlying causes of the problem. However they will neither develop nor implement solutions.

Analogous to industrial quality assurance

Many of the terms used to describe audit activities (quality assessment, quality evaluation, quality assurance, quality control) are coloured by the image of an industrial production line.

The inappropriateness of the analogy is that human well-being and the health care industry which deals with it are infinitely more complex than production lines. These involve a limited number of processes which are carried out in a fixed sequence; in health care a very large number of processes are available and the skill lies in selecting the appropriate ones in the correct order. Further, when a problem occurs in the production line the fault can often be remedied by adjusting the responsible machine. In health care effecting change is much more difficult because it often involves modifying the behaviour of health professionals (see Chapter 8).

Although not generally applicable, there is one area of medicine where industrial quality control methods are appropriate. A national quality control scheme for pathology laboratories was implemented in 1969 [31]. This involves the routine monitoring of the quality of clinical chemistry analyses in hospital laboratories. The scheme is successful because the product, chemical estimation, is easy to measure and the remedy, improved technique, relatively easy to implement.

Routine data collection

Several studies which routinely collect data on every patient attending a clinic over a period of years have been published under the banner of audit. Why they are unlikely to lead to improvements in the delivery of health care is clear from the audit cycle (Figure 2.4). Routine systems are not able to respond when the requirements for data change as the topic is refined; they will often not collect the data needed to identify the underlying causes of a problem. Even when allied to sophisticated computer systems the potential for audit is limited: *'we used to have lots of questions to which there were no answers. Now, with computers, there are lots of answers to which we haven't thought up the questions'* (Sir Peter Ustinov)[32]. Naturally, when routine data systems have been established for other purposes, they can provide a convenient way of getting some of the data needed for audit. However, for audit alone, the limited contribution these systems can make does not justify the time and effort required to develop them.

One defence of routine data collection systems is that audit can be carried out as a by-product of a system established for other purposes. Thus most of the commercial computer packages for audit will also run patient administration systems, manage waiting lists and theatre lists, and write discharge letters [33]. Each of these other activities presents its own difficulties, consuming time and energy while not advancing the aims of audit. These other activities are undoubtedly valuable in themselves but they are not audit. It is sometimes argued that these activities should be combined with audit because there is such an overlap in the data required for them. The reasoning behind this claim has been referred to as *'the fallacy of the common core of data'* [34]. Audit focuses on the way care is delivered to identify reasons for inadequate care. It investigates a very specific area of care, and collects detailed data on that area on a selected set of patients for a specified time. Patient administration systems collect more general information on all patients and continue doing so indefinitely.

Many hospitals have computer systems which contain data on patient characteristics, laboratory tests, discharge diagnoses, and prescribed drugs. These systems are often separate but can in theory be linked. The attractions of linking are obvious and official advice to clinicians is that linked data sets offer great scope for audit [35]. However the limitations of routine data systems apply with at least as much force to large hospital computer systems. Sophisticated computer systems bring with them a host of tasks which are unrelated to audit and its needs. Just because the system contains data on thousands of patients and involves sophisticated computer programming, this will not overcome shortcomings in the quality or relevance of the data. The problems of routine data collection are reviewed in more detail in Chapter 6.

SUMMARY

This chapter has outlined the essential features of audit and shown how the audit cycle guides the conduct of studies. From these discussions it is possible to identify the principles of good audit.

- *Primary aim is to improve the delivery of health care*
  The audit project should be designed so that effecting change is the intention from an early stage. Observing practice is common, and often interesting, but usually leads nowhere. Involvement in peripheral activities such as patient administration systems should be avoided.

- *Confidential*
  The findings of audit studies will often be revealed to interested groups including management, but the identity of medical staff and patients must always be completely confidential. If necessary the original data should be destroyed before findings are released.

- *Educational*
  The conduct of audit studies often has a general educational benefit in addition to the primary aim of effecting change in a specific area. Thus audit should be conducted in a supportive rather than a judgemental environment. Audit can also identify areas of educational need which, when dealt with, can lead to improvements in care.

- *Parsimonious*
  Resources for audit are limited so the simplest method should be used, the study should be run for the shortest possible time and only essential data should be collected. Ambitious data collection systems are costly, rigid, and thus inefficient for audit.

- *Focused*
  Audit should concentrate on the topics which will lead to the greatest improvements in health care. This will involve focusing on very specific aspects of care.

- *Seek the underlying cause*
  The key to effective audit is to determine the underlying causes of any deficiency in health care. This will enable a specific solution to be devised.

- *Flexible*
  The audit can evolve as data are collected which refine the nature of the problem. Allied to the need to search for the underlying cause, audit must be flexible.

● *Collaborative*
Audit studies will be more likely to achieve success if they have the enthusiastic support of all staff. A cardinal rule for achieving this is to involve everyone from the beginning and strive for a high level of commitment throughout the study.

● *Resourced*
Even a simple audit project will involve staff time for data collection, analysis, interpretation and the more difficult task of effecting change in the delivery of health care. Since good communication is fundamental to audit, additional time will have to be set aside for keeping colleagues informed.

● *Standards*
Audit involves comparing current practice against desirable standards of care. Standards should be objective and explicitly stated. The standards have to be attainable otherwise the findings of audit studies will be rejected as unrealistic.

● *Tactful*
Effecting change is the most difficult stage of audit, and should be handled with sensitivity and ingenuity.

● *Assessed*
Attempts to effect change may achieve only partial success, so it is important to assess the impact of any intervention. If insufficient change has been achieved then the audit cycle may have to be repeated.

REFERENCES

1. Baker R. Problem solving with audit in general practice. Br Med J 1990; 300: 378–80.
2. Shaw CD, Costain DW. Guidelines for medical audit: seven principles. Br Med J 1989; 299: 498–9.
3. Smith T. Medical audit: closing the feedback loop is vital. Br Med J 1990; 300: 65.
4. McKee CM, Lauglo M, Lessof L. Medical audit: a review. J Roy Soc Med 1989; 82: 474–8.
5. Royal College of General Practitioners. Quality in General Practice. London: Royal College of General Practitioners, 1985.

6. Royal College of Physicians. Medical audit: a first report. London: Royal College of Physicians, 1989.

7. Royal College of Surgeons. Guidelines to clinical audit in surgical practice. London: Royal College of Surgeons, 1989.

8. Chambers Twentieth Century Dictionary. Edinburgh: Constable, 1973.

9. Slee VN. In: Eisele CW, ed. The medical staff and the modern hospital. New York: McGraw Hill, 1967.

10. Ellis BW. How to set up an audit. Br Med J 1989; 298: 1635–7.

11. Heath DA. The appropriate use of diagnostic services: (xiii) Medical audit in clinical practice and medical education. Health Trends 1986; 18: 74–6.

12. Dixon N. Medical audit primer. Hampshire: Healthcare Quality Quest, 1991.

13. Fowkes FGR. Medical Audit Cycle. Med Educ 1982; 16: 228–38.

14. Hancock BD. Audit of major colorectal and biliary surgery to reduce rates of wound infection. Br Med J 1990; 301: 911–2.

15. Higgins AF, Lewis A, Noone P, Hole ML. Single and multiple dose cotrimoxazole and metronidazole in colorectal surgery. Br J Surg 1980; 67: 90–2.

16. Donabedian A. The quality of care: how can it be assessed? J Am Med Assoc 1988; 260: 1743–8.

17. Shaw CD. Criterion based audit. Br Med J 1990; 300: 649–51.

18. Shaw CD. Aspects of Audit: 5. Looking forward to audit. Br Med J 1980; i: 1509–11.

19. Standing Committee On Postgraduate Medical Education. Medical audit: the educational implications. London: SCOPME, 1989.

20. Buck N, Devlin HB, Lunn JN. Report of a confidential enquiry into perioperative deaths. London: Nuffield Provincial Hospital Trust, 1987.

21. Puntis JWL, Holden CE, Smallman S, Finkel Y, George RH, Booth IW. Staff training: a key factor in reducing intravascular catheter sepsis. Arch Dis Child 1990; 65: 335–7.

22. Department of Health. Medical Audit: Working Paper 6. London: HMSO, 1989.

23. Firth-Cozens J, Venning P. Audit officers: what are they up to? Br Med J 1991; 303: 631–2.

24. Cohen JM, Cohen MJ. Dictionary of modern quotations. London: Penguin, 1980.

25. Sharples PM, Storey A, Aynsley-Green A, Eyre JA. Avoidable factors contributing to death of children with head injury. Br Med J 1990; 300: 87–91.

26. Mitchell MW, Fowkes FGR. Audit reviewed: does feedback on performance change clinical behaviour? J R Coll Physicians London 1985; 19: 251–4.
27. Mugford M, Banfield P, O'Hanlon M. Effects of feedback of information on clinical practice: a review. Br Med J 1991; 303: 398–402.
28. Fisher RB, Dearden CH. Improving the care of patients with major trauma in the accident and emergency department. Br Med J 1990; 300: 1560–3.
29. Crombie IK, Davies HTO. The missing link in the audit cycle. Quality in Health Care 1993 (in press).
30. Pollock AV. The rise and fall of the random trial in surgery. Theor Surg 1989; 4: 163–70.
31. Whitehead T. Surveying the performance of pathological laboratories. In: McLachlan G, ed. A Question of Quality. London: Oxford University Press, 1976: 97–117.
32. Green J. A dictionary of contemporary quotations. London: Pan, 1982.
33. Tyndall R, Kennedy S, Naylor S, Pajack F. Computers in medical audit. London: Royal Society of Medicine, 1990.
34. Crombie IK, Davies HTO. Computers in audit: servants or sirens? Br Med J 1991; 303: 403–4.
35. Department of Health. Medical audit: guidance for hospital clinicians on the use of computers. London: HMSO, 1990.

3

Management of Audit

Audit involves people. No-one practices in a vacuum; even single-handed practitioners interact with colleagues in referring patients and use support services. The results of audit often have implications for colleagues and other professional groups and, to be effective, audit needs to take account of their beliefs, concerns and motivations. This chapter begins by reviewing strategies for introducing audit, to allay the concerns that are often felt.

The collaborative nature of audit brings additional problems. Success depends on nurturing good working relations and promoting individual development. Thus this chapter also focuses on the management of groups.

INTRODUCING AUDIT

Clinicians can have strong and opposing reactions to audit. Some may welcome it enthusiastically, while others may feel threatened and avoid involvement. The primary aim of audit, improving the delivery of health care, implies the management of change in professional behaviour to which there may be resistance if not hostility. Yet to be successful audit has to have the active support of all those involved. To achieve this audit needs to be introduced slowly and sensitively.

Attitudes to audit

Audit can be threatening because of its potential to reveal deficiencies in health care services. Clinicians may fear that results will portray previous patient care as inadequate, and thus undermine their professional reputation. Yet maintaining and enhancing this reputation is central to work motivation. Clinicians may also anticipate that, by criticising established medical practice, audit will undermine confidence in care regimes, without offering suitable alternatives. Thus audit can simultaneously threaten reputation, work satisfaction and professional security. Some may feel that if deficiencies in care are identified, changes may be imposed. Audit may thus be seen as an attempt to curtail clinical freedom; *'I began to have visions of increasing bureaucracy and interference with clinical practice'* [1].

Audit may give rise to concern because the term carries the implication of *'numerical review by an outside investigator directed at, among other things, the prevention of fraud'* [2]. Thus clinicians may view audit as a precursor to expenditure cuts, suspecting it to be a means of *'ferreting out embezzlers ... another fiendish Government device to save money'* [3].

Many clinicians are not opposed to audit, but welcome it. This is not without difficulties: enthusiasts may have unrealistic expectations about its potential to solve practice problems, anticipating that it will provide new medical insights, improve patient care and simultaneously enhance their own professional standing. Such enthusiasm is positive but must be tempered if it is not to result in loss of motivation when audit falls short of these expectations. Strong enthusiasm may also threaten others who approach audit with caution. It may further confirm suspicions that those involved in audit emerge as either winners or losers.

Managing responses to audit

If audit elicits any of the responses described above, it will be avoided and resisted. Encouraging participation in, and commitment to audit depends upon recognizing and managing these different responses. Simple principles can be used to guide the management of audit groups to constructive and productive working relations:

- Identify current review activities.
- Acknowledge and address participants' concerns.
- Emphasise confidentiality.
- Emphasise local control.
- Set modest aims and objectives.
- Emphasise the value of present and past practice.
- Associate audit with enhanced professional standing.

To overcome the idea that audit is a recent unwanted imposition, the types of review activities which are currently undertaken, such as case presentations, could be discussed. Although sometimes overlooked, audit is not a new activity in Britain, and there are many examples of successful worthwhile studies which have been completed (see Chapter 1).

Early reassurance may encourage participation and prevent later withdrawal. This will be promoted if participants feel valued and realise that they will not be judged or censured. Continued commitment is most likely when all members are kept fully informed and constructive comment and debate is actively facilitated.

One important feature of audit is that it is not done by others, but is carried out by the group for the benefit of the group, and is under local control. Threat is reduced when participants feel they are involved in a step-by-step process over which they have control. Audit begins with exploratory information gathering which enables participants to decide whether they wish to continue the audit. Potential policy or practice implications should only emerge when more detailed findings are reviewed. Participants will be reassured by the knowledge that audit data will be fully discussed before any changes need to be considered.

When change is recommended it is important to avoid attributing blame for previous failures: *'if people are afraid of each other within an organisation, if information can be used to harm someone, or if managers blame people for failures built into the process of work, then real quality improvement can easily grind to a halt'* [4]. Instead it should be emphasised that in general work has been of a high standard and audit provides an opportunity for further improvement. It is a way of generating reliable evaluative information which can enhance professional effectiveness through practitioners' own decisions to maintain or modify practice.

Attention to colleagues' potential responses to audit enables the process to be portrayed as an 'all-win' opportunity to enhance service delivery, personal effectiveness and reputation. Ignoring these responses or managing them badly may lead to conflict, apathy, trivialisation and sabotage of the audit process.

The early meetings

The possible anxieties which group members may have about audit need to be tackled early. Coping with these and the diverse views on audit may occupy several meetings. These discussions could lead to a group consensus on the approach that it wishes to take to audit. They could involve discussions of the characteristics of audit (see Chapter 2), and identify what the group hopes to achieve through it.

A common problem in planning audit is to get side-tracked into discussions of subjects which are better dealt with later. Some of these are:

- Topics for audit.
- Methods of audit.
- Minimum data set.
- Computing equipment.

There is a natural temptation to want to identify topics, design projects, and begin data collection. This may give the illusion that progress is being made, but, because of insufficient planning, the projects may be poor and lead to disillusionment. A brief inspection of Chapters 4 to 7 of this book should demonstrate that these are complex issues which will take time to resolve. These chapters also explain how the problems are well within the group's competence to solve. For example, from Chapter 4 a list of topics for audit could be prepared, so that the group can more quickly agree that finding them is not a problem and can be safely postponed. Perhaps the most seductive and least useful distraction is the attempt to identify the minimum data set which will enable many audits to be carried out. It does not exist. Chapter 6 reviews the types of data needed for audit, showing how the data for each study are likely to be unique, and how, even within a study the essential data may change as progress is made round the audit cycle.

A MANAGEMENT DISASTER

Audit studies need careful planning and management. An example, based on the experience of one of the authors a number of years ago, illustrates what can go wrong when a study is poorly planned and managed. Some of the details have been changed to ensure the confidentiality of those involved, but the mistakes and their consequences are real.

The background

Senior clinical staff in surgery were concerned that prostatectomy was not being managed as well as it could be. Their concerns were that some patients had unnecessary delays in the operation which could compromise its success, and also that some operations were unnecessary. They decided to audit their practice to identify the reasons for delays and to assess the appropriateness of the operations carried out. At an early planning meeting it emerged that surgeons in another teaching hospital had similar concerns, so a joint study was proposed in the hope that a comparison between the centres would shed light on deficiencies of care.

The study

Several meetings were held at which the study aims and design were discussed. At any one meeting there were usually two professors, at least six consultants, two senior registrars and a statistician. The study took many meetings to design, but enthusiasm was maintained and every effort was taken to ensure that any data item which might be relevant had been identified. A questionnaire was developed and a pilot study conducted, in which a senior registrar at each centre was delegated to abstract the data from 100 case-notes. This took much longer than anticipated and data were only collected at one centre. Progress was temporarily halted because the nominal secretary to the group had become heavily involved in other activities. Although the data were eventually entered into a computer they were never analysed. The main study never took place, nor did any further meetings, not because the project was ever formally abandoned but because enthusiasm had finally run out.

Why did it go wrong?

This study failed for a variety of reasons. The committee which designed the study was too big with no clear leadership. The meetings it held were largely unstructured. Each lasted two to three hours, but it was often difficult to identify which decisions had been taken, so that some were retaken on subsequent occasions. Because committee members were often unsure who had been allocated responsibility for particular tasks, appropriate actions were often not taken.

The resulting study design was poor. A formal protocol, which could have been evaluated critically, was never written and the practicability of the study was not assessed. The project aims evolved into an unexciting compromise between the conflicting views of the committee. As the aims changed new data items were added but none were ever removed so that too much complex data were collected.

The management of the study was equally unsatisfactory. There was no mechanism for assessing progress, and no attempts were made to identify delays. Little thought was given to the collection, processing and analysis of the data. In the event, data collection was delegated to unwilling senior registrars. Because the final data set was so large and complex, and the project aims ill-defined and unexciting, the analysis was never carried out.

GROUP MANAGEMENT IN AUDIT

'A committee is a cul de sac down which ideas are lured and then quietly strangled' (Sir Barnett Cocks)[5].

The disaster story described above highlights the importance of group management in audit. Ineffective group management led to poorly defined objectives and inadequate planning. The timetabling of the project was unrealistic, responsibilities were not clearly allocated and some staff only participated reluctantly. Individual talents can be harnessed to create a well organized and productive group, but this requires attention to members' concerns and motivations; and an understanding of the effects of group influences upon decision-making.

Managing audit meetings

Clear, timely communication is vital to collaborative working. Group members need to understand the objectives of particular meetings and complete the necessary preparation. However there is no single best way to organise and run meetings, as this depends on what the meeting is intended to achieve.

Traditional committee management procedures are best when the timing and coordination of work is a priority. They often exhibit several features:

- Tight time control.
- Agendas.
- Action minutes.
- Strong leadership.

Meetings need to run to time; distinctions have to be drawn between issues requiring immediate attention because of external deadlines and those which can be considered over longer periods. This can be encouraged by agendas circulated well in advance. Action between meetings depends upon participants understanding what others expect of them and what decisions they can and should act upon. This can be prompted by the circulation of action minutes which identify tasks for named members. This type of meeting needs strong, although not dictatorial, leadership: *'good leaders are not authoritarian, nor are they shrinking violets. They believe in forging consensus and then helping everybody share in the implementation'* [6].

However, these control procedures may be counter productive when objectives and plans are evolving. Bureaucratic or authoritarian management may suppress creativity [7, 8]. These management approaches discourage participation by emphasising rule-following. By concentrating decision-making in a few key individuals they limit collective responsibility. For example, the productivity of a meeting called to generate new ideas could be seriously undermined by the constraints of committee procedure. Optimum control procedures depend upon the stage of the audit process and the commitment of group members.

Fostering cooperation

Cooperation and understanding cannot be taken for granted within groups. Constructive interaction often needs to be nurtured. This requires skilled contributions, especially from those who hold leadership responsibilities (such as chairpersons). Key activities include:

- Listening carefully to others' ideas and reservations.
- Encouraging and praising others' contributions.
- Summarising and clarifying progress during discussions.
- Identifying similarities and compromises during disagreements.
- Mediating between those with different perspectives.
- Relieving tension through humour or creating breaks.
- Managing participation so that everyone is involved.

A socially skilled chairperson may sometimes perform many of these functions for a group. But, more commonly, effective meetings depend upon the majority of participants contributing to these management activities.

An important advantage of a person-orientated approach to managing meetings is that it tends to minimise attention- and control-seeking behaviour. Nevertheless, groups often have to deal with the expression of anxieties and unmet needs. Those who continue to feel threatened by audit may resist sharing control or block progress. Some may seek attention from the group by being aggressive towards others or may try to focus proceedings upon their particular interests. Those who feel anxious in group meetings may withdraw or divert attention towards other topics. Common disruptive problems include members who:

- Devalue others' expertise and work practices.
- Reject others' ideas and proposals without acknowledging their value.
- Blame or intimidate others.
- Distract discussion into personal interests or previously discussed issues.
- Block progress by refusing to compromise.
- Display cynicism or indifference.
- Withdraw by non-attendance or non-participation.
- Encourage conflict between others.

Ignoring these difficulties may be effective when the issues involved are trivial or the group's life is likely to be short. However, in the longer term they are likely to result in reduced motivation or the fragmentation of groups.

Resolving these interpersonal problems involves the investment of time in exploration and negotiation. A first step towards confronting interpersonal problems is to observe and describe what is happening to disrupt group productivity. Explicit acknowledgement of the problems may be enough to promote self-discipline amongst members. Beyond this it may be possible to discuss conflicts of interests, fears, concerns and feelings which are generating destructive interaction. These discussions may be easier in smaller meetings between key protagonists. Whatever the setting, compromise, accommodation and cooperative collaboration are likely to be facilitated if group members are able to acknowledge one another's concerns.

Managing group decision-making

Good decision-making may be elusive even in cooperative and productive groups. In groups, individuals tend to value the opinion of others and to seek agreement. This can persuade some to adopt or tolerate viewpoints which they previously rejected. Conformity prompted by a desire for others' approval may only be temporary and members may return to their previous perspective outside the group. This may erode their commitment to the group's decisions, undermining group plans and delaying progress.

It is possible to shield group members from the pressure to agree with others when decisions have to be made. Without this protection the group loses access to viewpoints which individuals refrain from expressing because of their potential social costs. For example, if someone feels that their evaluation of the group's proposals will create problems in an important alliance or sour relationships with a powerful figure who controls valuable resources, they may conform without conviction. The loss of such perspectives on the group's activities reduces its capacity for thoroughly considered decision-making.

Such difficulties can be avoided if decision-making is carefully managed. The following guidelines can help:

- Articulate clearly defined objectives when making plans.
- Sample individual opinions separately from group discussions.
- Schedule time to debate proposals critically.
- Encourage the expression of minority viewpoints.
- Invite outside consultation and evaluation.
- Evaluate and reconsider at each stage of a project.

Encouraging debate and evaluation, and fostering personal commitment rather than tolerant acceptance, are crucial prerequisites to effective audit.

Fostering creativity

Creative participation in an audit group is not easily achieved. It depends upon persuading each member that they have something valuable to contribute, and acknowledging that creative ideas sometimes appear unusual or misguided when first considered. Otherwise members may fear rejection or ridicule, and wait for others to take the lead. This can lead to low participation, reduced commitment to the group's activities and the loss of potentially fruitful ideas.

A number of techniques have been developed to help establish a creative group climate. Their essential ingredient is that the generation of ideas is separated from their critical evaluation. Brainstorming is probably the best known of these. A facilitator encourages other group members to say the first thing that comes into their head in response to a specific word or question. These are listed on a blackboard or flip chart. All ideas are taken seriously and none are evaluated or modified at this stage. Thus in thinking about improving patient satisfaction with consultations, ideas such as 'waiting room videos', 'doubling consultation length' or 'financial compensation for long waiting times' would all be equally welcome. Brainstorming can take as little as 20 minutes. It enables ideas to be shared without criticism, leading to a more relaxed group atmosphere. It is also likely to result in a list of potential ideas, identifying alternative ways of looking at a problem. However, it does not provide a mechanism for evaluating these ideas.

The 'nominal group' is a procedure for maximising the generation of ideas, and managing their evaluation, in face-to-face group meetings [9]. Before discussion, members are asked to write down suggestions. These individual contributions are then publicly recorded with each member offering one idea in turn until all are listed. At this stage the group begins the more practical task of evaluating ideas jointly. A series of specific evaluative criteria are agreed (for example, clarity, clinical importance, expense and practicality) and members silently consider each idea in terms of these criteria. Each idea could, for example, be rated out of ten on each criterion. The scores for each idea can be summed to give an indication of overall acceptability. The highest scoring idea is selected for further discussion. This technique protects creative thinking and also enables the group to evaluate ideas in a way that minimises group influences.

SUMMARY

This chapter has emphasised the importance of organising and managing groups to carry out audit.

Audit may be opposed because it is viewed as:

- Imposed from outside.
- A threat to clinical freedom.
- Primarily a cost cutting exercise.

Resistance to audit can be minimised by emphasising:

- Present high levels of staff competence.
- That audit is under local control.
- Confidentiality of all details.
- That audit is an opportunity for staff development.

The way in which a meeting is managed depends on its purpose. When the meeting is concerned with the timing and coordination of actions, it needs to:

- Be tightly controlled.
- Keep to a fixed agenda.
- Produce action minutes.

The generation of ideas and the development of study design needs to:

- Encourage participation.
- Encourage discussion.
- Separate the generation of ideas from their assessment.

Good decision making can be elusive in groups, even when they are well managed. Strategies to facilitate decision-making include:

- Define clear objectives.
- Encourage expression of minority views.
- Sample views away from meetings.
- Canvas opinions of outside experts.
- Reassess project at each stage.

REFERENCES

1. Godfrey R. Called to account: a consultant physician. Lancet 1989; i: 606–7.
2. Shaw CD. Aspects of Audit: 1. The background. Br Med J 1980; i: 1256–8.
3. Lilleyman JS. Called to account: a haematologist. Lancet 1989; i: 545–6.
4. Berwick DM, Enthoven A, Bunker JP. Quality management in the NHS: the doctor's role—I. Br Med J 1992; 304: 235–9.
5. Green J. A dictionary of contemporary quotations. London: Pan, 1982.
6. Macmillan L, Pringle M. Practice managers and practice management. Br Med J 1992; 304: 1672–4.
7. White P, Lippitt R. Leader behaviour and member reaction in three social climates. In: Cartwright D, Zander A, eds. Group Dynamics; Research and Theory. 3rd edn. London: Tavistock, 1968: 318–35.
8. Hersey P, Blanchard KH. Management of organisational behaviour: utilizing human resources. New Jersey: Prentice Hall, Engelwood Cliffs, 1982.
9. Delbecq AL, Van de Ven AH, Gustafson DH. Group techniques for program planning: a guide to nominal and Delphi processes. Illinois: Scott Foresman, 1975.

4

Topics for Audit

Topics for audit are virtually unlimited. The White Paper definition indicated that audit should cover *'the procedures used for diagnosis and treatment, the use of resources and the resulting outcome and quality of life for the patient'*. In short all aspects of medical care are suitable and even a brief inspection of the literature will disclose an abundance of topics from all specialties. This chapter reviews the areas of medical care which can be audited and presents methods for identifying fruitful topics.

The profusion of topics brings with it the problem of selection. Experience in the United States [1] and Britain [2] is that finding topics is easy; the difficulty lies in selecting those which are worthwhile. This chapter identifies criteria for evaluating topics and develops methods for selecting them.

AREAS FOR AUDIT

To review topics for audit it is useful to arrange them in categories. A popular subdivision, attributed to the American theoretician Donabedian, suggests that there are three types of question which we can ask of health care: what facilities are there? what was done to the patient? and what was the result for the patient? These three questions identify the principal categories for audit topics: structure, process, and outcome.

Table 4.1   *Examples of topics for audit*

Areas	Examples
Structure	
Premises	Structural integrity; clinic space; waiting space for patients; operating theatres
Furniture	Beds; chairs; trolleys
Staffing	Numbers of doctors, nurses, paramedical staff, and clerical staff; training, experience; continuing education
Diagnostic equipment	Available; working; e.g. X-ray machines, opthalmoscopes, peak flow meters, defibrillators
Access to support services	Diagnostic services, e.g. immunology, microbiology, clinical chemistry; support services, e.g. physiotherapy, clinical psychology
Process	
Referral	Quality of referral letter; appropriateness of referral; who is not sending patients, but should be; size of waiting list and the time patients have to wait; reasons for failure to attend
Admission	Delays in admission; delays occurring before the patient arrives at the appropriate specialty; drugs recorded on admission
Investigations	Appropriateness and quality of investigations; impact on clinical management; relevant investigations not carried out
Diagnosis	Accuracy; timeliness
General treatment	Appropriateness; timeliness
Nursing care	Frequency of monitoring patients; delay in responding to calls; timeliness of drug administration
Drugs	Adherence to formulary; dosage and administration; drug interactions; contraindications
Screening	Cervical and breast cancers; neonatal
Disease prevention	Immunization and vaccination; health promotion
Techniques	Surgical; anaesthetic; psychotherapy; rehabilitation
Quality of case-notes	Initial booking adequate; clinical problems clearly set out; course of illness and management documented; notes signed
Communication	Between senior and junior staff; between specialties; requests for services
Hotel facilities	Food; day rooms; access to newspapers, shopping
Discharge	Unnecessary hospital stay; rationalisation of drugs; quality and timeliness of discharge letters; appropriateness of follow-up appointments and

Table 4.1   *(continued)*

Areas	Examples
	onward referral; existence of a discharge policy; account taken of personal circumstances; contact with social services

Outcome

Areas	Examples
Mortality	Post-surgical; intensive care; perinatal; chronic diseases, e.g. diabetes, asthma, hypertension
Disease state	Cure; remission; improvement
Symptom control	Post-operative pain; joint pain (rheumatic); fits (epilepsy)
Residual disability	Physical impairment; emotional health; social functioning; cognitive functioning; quality of life
Proxy measures	Blood glucose (diabetes); respiratory function (asthma)
Unwanted outcomes	Post-operative wound infection; pressure sores; falls in hospital; nosocomial infection; procedural problems (e.g. infusion, transfusion); adverse effects of drugs, anaesthesia, surgery
Indirect measures	Unscheduled surgery; unscheduled admission to intensive care; re-admission to hospital, re-appearance at out-patients; time off work; frequency of subsequent GP contacts; number of subsequent drugs

Patient satisfaction

Areas	Examples
Access	Availability of services; distance to clinic; waiting time at clinic; out-of-hours service
Information	On diagnosis; on treatment; on long-term outcome
Clinical staff	Apparent competence; politeness; dress; interest in patient; attention to psychosocial problems; continuity in care
Facilities	Waiting rooms; access to toilets, shops and telephones; chiropody service; smoke-free lounge

Table 4.1 gives an outline of the areas in these categories which could be audited, and for each area examples of topics are listed. Patient satisfaction has been added to this table because it is sufficiently important to be highlighted, even though it overlaps with outcome.

Structure

Structure refers to the buildings, equipment, and staff involved in health care. This includes hospitals, health centres, community clinics and all the equipment contained in them. One of the major concerns when the National Health Service was formed in 1948 was to remedy the evident deficiencies in buildings and equipment. These early deficiencies were largely resolved, but some problems remain. A report on genitourinary medicine clinics described conditions reminiscent of the 19th Century: *'appalling adapted premises in basements and yards ... in cramped conditions food and beverages were seen being prepared on the bench used for infected secretions'* [3]. In part the problems arose because of an increase in the number of difficult and time-consuming cases of viral infection. Advances in medical science can also lead to unsatisfactory health care; equipment which was adequate in the past could be outmoded today. The most obvious example is the rapid development of computing in medicine; a survey of cervical screening services provided by district health authorities found that 60% had inadequate software packages [4].

Structure also includes the number of staff involved in delivering health care and their levels of training and experience. The balance between senior and junior doctors, nurses and paramedical staff, technical and clerical staff is not always optimal; an audit of the usage of operating theatre time found that understaffing was the largest single cause of under-utilisation [5]. The level of experience of the staff may also be an issue as avoidable errors are sometimes made by unsupervised junior staff [6].

Remedying deficiencies in structure can be difficult: it may be more a matter for the health authority than the clinician. However this does not mean that there is no point in auditing structure. Demonstrating that inadequacies are due to insufficient resources can be a powerful argument for more. Following the publication of the survey of the genitourinary medicine clinics an extra £130 million was allocated for the following year and the health minister responsible commented *'these services have been neglected in too many places for too long'* [7].

Process

The most common type of audit is that of *process*, examining what was done to the patient in terms of investigations, diagnosis and treatment to determine how well the patient was managed. Audits of process assess whether the quality of care given was as good as could be achieved in the circumstances. It is thus complementary to audits of structure which investigate whether the resources available for the management of the patients are satisfactory.

A good example of an audit of process is the management of patients referred for invasive cardiovascular investigation and intervention [8]. The patient group is easily defined and identified, and criteria of good care, the interval between investigation and intervention, can be measured. The audit found that the *'response to emergency referral is inadequate'*, and *'the waiting time to routine investigation and revascularisation is prolonged and seems to be worsening.'* This type of audit focuses on the management of patients with a particular condition, asking questions like:

- What was done?
- How well was it done?
- What should have been done?

One way to answer these questions is to compare the actual management of the patient against an agreed management protocol to identify aspects of care which were neglected, carried out too late, or were unnecessary.

Treatment can also be assessed by focusing not on specific patient groups, but on the type of treatment itself. Compliance with treatment and the prescription of contraindicated drugs have frequently been audited. Selecting the drugs to investigate is greatly simplified by texts such as *Safer Prescribing* [9] which list several hundred potential drug problems. Many institutions now have formularies of recommended drugs to encourage the prescribing of effective drugs and to reduce costs. But the development of new drug therapies presents continuing scope for audit, of which thrombolytic therapy is an obvious one. For example, Morgan and colleagues [10] describe how local guidelines can be implemented to balance cost and clinical indications for the drugs streptokinase, alteplase and anistreplase.

Individual procedures and investigations can be audited in the same way as treatments, asking questions like:

- Was it justified?
- How well was it carried out?
- Were the results acted upon?

The Royal College of Radiologists' concerns about *'the increasingly expensive and often inefficient use that is being made of diagnostic facilities'* led them to set up a working party in 1975 [11]. An initial survey of pre-operative chest X-rays revealed that many were carried out unnecessarily and even clinically significant findings often had no influence on patient management. Guidelines were produced and subsequent interventions successfully reduced the frequency with which chest X-rays were used.

Audit which looks at the use of resources is not restricted to investigations and procedures, but includes the use of beds, operating theatres, utilisation of staff and the organisation of out-patient clinics. One survey of patients attending a general medical out-patient clinic found that over one quarter of patients were also attending another clinic for the same or a related problem, in most cases in a different hospital [12]. The authors pointed out that reviewing follow-up out-patient attendances could *'not only ensure a more effective service overall but would also save patients and their relatives from inconvenience.'* Although service efficiency is primarily the concern of resource management, it is also a legitimate subject for audit because inefficient resource use can sometimes result in poor care. For example patients attending more than one out-patient clinic will increase the length of time other patients have to wait, and could also be over-investigated or prescribed contraindicated drugs.

Communication between professionals is another fruitful source of topics for audit. Problems can occur through absence of communication as well as through a mishap in the process. An audit of adolescent self-harm patients showed that over one-third were discharged *'without specific psychiatric consultation or other follow-up'*, and concluded *'doctors working in accident and emergency should be encouraged to liaise with child psychiatrists before discharging such patients'* [13]. A survey of the communication of necropsy reports found that only 59% of the reports were seen by the consultant responsible for the patient and only 47% of the GPs were informed [14]. Communication is worth particular emphasis because interfaces are so numerous in patient care. For example Figure 4.1 illustrates some of the many groups who are involved in in-patient care: the referring physician, the specialties in addition to those responsible for patient care, and those responsible for the patient after discharge. Many other support services could be added to the diagram, but the opportunities for communication failures are clear even with this simple representation of care.

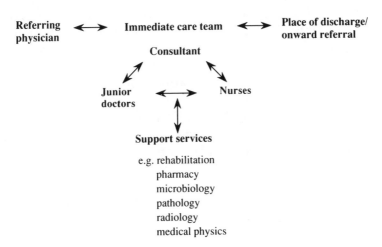

Figure 4.1 *Some professional interfaces in the care of an in-patient*

Outcome

The most important question for medical care is how successful was it? The types of questions asked in audits of *outcome* of treatment are:

● Did the patient experience the expected benefit?
● Were there any adverse effects?

Audit of outcome is acknowledged to be the most difficult because of the problems of measuring the consequences of treatment. In recognition of this over $30 million was allocated for research into measures of outcome in the United States in 1990 [15].

Measuring outcome can be straightforward, when, as in antibiotics for gonorrhoea, the treatment produces a complete cure. Similarly it may be easy when the outcome focuses not on the benefits of treatment but on unexpected adverse events, such as rebleeding of peptic ulcer or frequent fits in epilepsy. Other adverse events which have been studied include post-operative wound infection and adverse drug reactions.

Death is the most extreme adverse event. Two of the best known audits, the confidential enquiries into maternal deaths [16] and peri-operative deaths [17] were primarily concerned with avoidable mortality. A range of conditions in which the occurrence of death may indicate inadequate care has been identified [18]. These include deaths from cervical cancer, acute respiratory infection, asthma, appendicitis, inguinal hernia, cholecystitis, and pernicious anaemia. Death can be a useful measure for these serious conditions, or for major operations which carry a high risk. It is of little relevance for less serious conditions like minor trauma or the common infectious diseases.

Audit of outcome can be especially difficult for many chronic diseases, such as rheumatoid arthritis. The result of a successful treatment may only be to arrest or slow down disease progression; for example in rheumatoid arthritis 'there is an increased mortality and substantial functional decline in patients with RA even if they receive apparently optimal treatment with antirheumatic drugs' [19]. Destruction of major joints or death can be used as outcome [20] but these will only be relevant to a minority of patients with severe long-standing disease. Symptom control (morning stiffness, pain and swelling in joints) can be used for most patients, although it is not certain that controlling symptoms is the same as treating the underlying condition. An alternative approach is to use measures of levels of disability and psychological well-being. These type of outcomes need more sophisticated measuring instruments to overcome the problems inherent in subjective patient reports. Reliable and valid measures of these outcomes have been developed, and these are covered in Chapter 7. Using and interpreting some of these measures requires skill and experience, and thought might be given to collaboration with a sociologist or psychologist.

In some conditions it is possible to use biochemical or physical measurements as proxies for outcome. For example, an audit of the management of diabetes in general practice [21] focused on blood glucose levels. The audit found that standards of care achieved (19% with satisfactory blood glucose) fell far short of the target (90%). Other conditions where proxy measures could be used are obesity, hypertension, and familial hyper-cholesterolaemia. Physiological measures used as proxies have two characteristics: they are closely associated with the disease under study, and successful treatment of the disease changes the level of the physiological measure. It is important that the proxy measure really is a predictor of disease state. Fries [22] reviewed proxy measures of arthritis, concluding that some (erythrocyte sedimentation rate and latex fixation titres) were much poorer measures of disease status and patient well-being than others (joint counts and haemoglobin level).

Process or Outcome?

The argument whether to audit process (easier), or outcome (more relevant), has concerned theoreticians for many years. However it is not always clear whether a topic should be classified as process or outcome; for example an investigation of the availability of transplantable organs from brain stem dead donors in intensive care units [23] could be considered *outcome* when viewed from the perspective of the providing unit, but *process* from the perspective of the receiving unit. Further, audits which begin by investigating unsatisfactory outcomes will often find that the underlying reason for unsatisfactory care lies in a failure of process. In the sense that audit is concerned with remedying these defective processes most audits of outcome could also be classified as audits of process.

A common assumption is that if the structure and process are satisfactory then good outcome is assured. However the relationship between process and outcome can be weak. One study of the management of hypertension found that several aspects of process (e.g. the quality of the medical history, the initial physical examination and laboratory tests) were not associated with good outcome [24]. There are many aspects of process which could be investigated but only a few of them may make the difference between good and poor outcome. The maxim *if it ain't broke don't fix it*, translates naturally from mechanical maintenance to become *if there isn't a problem don't audit it*. Thus it is not a question of whether it is better to audit process or outcome, but of focusing on important problems of whichever kind.

Patient satisfaction

Many audit studies have focused on the extent to which patients are satisfied with the treatment they have received. Patient satisfaction is strictly a type of outcome measure, but because of its significance it merits a section to itself. The importance of the patients' views on the delivery of care was emphasised in the 1989 White Paper, and has been strengthened by the issue of the Patient's Charter in 1991. Surveys of patient views can identify ways in which the service can be improved; one study of patients attending a genitourinary clinic found strong support for more flexible attendance arrangements and for evening openings [25]. These studies may also highlight areas of medical practice which need reassessment. Schofield and colleagues found that although women with severe pre-operative symptoms expressed satisfaction with their hysterectomy, those with less severe symptoms were less satisfied, leading to doubts about the value of the operation for such women [26].

There is more to good outcome than patient impressions: *'satisfaction is clearly only one dimension of outcome and does not necessarily reflect the quality of technical aspects of care—badly treated patients with poor medical outcomes may still feel satisfied'* [27]. However there are also good clinical reasons for being concerned with patient satisfaction. Compliance with therapy and the likelihood of patients showing up for repeat appointments are not surprisingly related to patient satisfaction [28]. Patient dissatisfaction may also reflect genuine deficiencies in care. Audits of patient satisfaction share the aim of other types of audit, to improve the delivery of health care, either by improving patient compliance or by dealing with problems the patients have identified.

Patient satisfaction is not an all or nothing phenomenon, but has many determinants [29, 30]. These are listed in Table 4.1 under four major headings: access; information; clinical staff; and facilities. One of the major problems of assessing patient satisfaction is the halo effect: patients typically report very high levels of satisfaction [31]. Assessing subjective states is far from easy, and requires sensitive, sophisticated measures. These measures are discussed in more detail in Chapter 7.

DECIDING WHAT TO AUDIT

The profusion of potential topics for audit brings with it the problem of selection. The time for audit is limited and even small projects may take several months to complete. If poor topics are chosen, time will be wasted and enthusiasm for audit will quickly be lost. Topics for audit could be selected by informal discussions between colleagues on those areas where health care may be less than optimal. This is likely to identify some worthwhile topics but equally will throw up some which are either wholly impracticable or turn out to be of only minor importance whereas many important topics may be overlooked.

A rational procedure for choosing topics is needed. Table 4.2 shows the steps involved in selecting a good topic for audit. Essentially a portfolio of potential topics is drawn up, from which, in discussion with colleagues, those of most clinical importance are selected. To be sure that the list of topics is likely

Table 4.2   *Deciding what to audit*

Draw up list of potential topics
- Agree approach to topic identification
- Discuss areas topics to be drawn from
- Construct portfolio

Select most important topics
- Agree method for setting priorities
- Agree criteria
- Assign priorities

Assess practicability
- Agree criteria
- Assess in theory
- Assess through small study

to contain clinically important ones a systematic approach to topic identification needs to be followed. Similarly a formal method of assessing clinical importance is required, if only to resolve disputes between clinicians about what is important. Finally the feasibility of each potential topic is assessed so that the overall judgement of priority is a balance between clinical importance and practicability. A more detailed description of the methods which can be used to carry out these steps is given in the following sections.

Identifying potential topics

Topics can be suggested from a variety of sources:

- Clinical experience.
- Case-note review.
- Literature review.
- Necropsy reports.
- Survey.
- Comparisons between centres.

Perhaps the easiest and most important source is clinical experience. It is likely to provide topics which are relevant to local circumstances and which at least some of the members of the audit group are concerned about. Locally relevant topics can also be identified by reviewing case-notes to identify aspects of care where there may be deficiencies. The emphasis of the review is on generating ideas rather than describing patient management in detail. Case-note review can also be used as a method of audit (see Chapter 6), but this requires more information on more cases than is necessary for topic identification. The temptation to dig too deeply should be resisted until it has been decided that the topic is suitable for a full scale audit.

Many of the topics reported on by other groups in the same specialty will have wider relevance, so that a literature review could be useful. This view has led several authors and two of the Royal Colleges to publish lists of topics for audit [20, 32–34]. Topics like appropriateness of investigations and treatment, delay in receiving treatment, length of stay in hospital, referral to support services, and communication between hospital and general practice can be audited in most hospital specialties.

Necropsies are an often overlooked but potentially rich source of topics for audit. A joint report from three of the Royal Colleges entitled *The Autopsy and Audit* indicates the scope for good topics from this source: *'much can be learned about the living from the study of the dead'* [35]. There may be potential for audit studies to prevent deaths by focusing on the reasons for lesions being missed.

Lastly a survey of the management of all patients seen over some period, such as six months or one year, can be carried out. This is undoubtedly a successful method of identifying topics; for example a survey of emergency admissions with abdominal pain found *'a need to review the management of ruptured aortic aneurism and perforated peptic ulcer, the methods of diagnosis of appendicitis, particularly in young females and the factors that determine the duration of stay of patients suffering from NSAP'* [36]. However the costs of carrying out surveys can be considerable and a common finding of those who have carried out surveys is that they took much more time and effort than had been anticipated [28]. Although a successful method for identifying topics, it is questionable whether surveys are efficient.

An important part of the process of identifying topics is that all of the members of the audit group should contribute. This will increase the number of topics identified and encourage everyone to feel involved in this the first stage of the audit cycle. Techniques to foster creativity were reviewed in Chapter 3.

Evaluating topics

As with many other stages of audit, evaluating topics is a group activity so that care needs to be taken to ensure that a genuine consensus is reached. Chapter 3 reviewed the principles for achieving this. Topics should be selected because the group feels they present clinically important problems which it is confident can be tackled successfully. General interest in a topic is insufficient: Baker [2] describes an audit of the management of hypertension begun out of curiosity. The initial findings were well received and no action was taken. It was only when a second survey three years later showed that the percentage of hypertensives not seen in the preceding year had doubled, that it was resolved to try to improve the management of hypertension.

Table 4.3 presents criteria which can be used to assess the suitability of a topic for audit. Clinical concern is undoubtedly the most important; the audit group are unlikely to develop sufficient enthusiasm to change their practice if they consider a topic to be of no clinical relevance. Such concern may arise from known differences in approaches to management. The management of transient ischaemic attacks is a case in point; the patients of some neurologists almost always underwent angiography, but those of other neurologists almost never did [37]. The frequency of carotid surgery also varied from 0% to 25%. Procedures which carry a high risk can give rise to clinical concern. The Lothian surgical audit [38] found evidence for avoidable post-operative mortality following vascular surgery, which was reduced when the operations were conducted only by specialist vascular surgeons. The difficulties posed by the long term management of chronic conditions increases the like-

Table 4.3   *Criteria for assessing topics*

Clinical concern
- Wide variation in clinical practice
- Major changes recently
- High risk procedures
- Conditions requiring rapid diagnosis or treatment
- Achievable benefits not achieved
- Complex or difficult management
- Involves other specialties

Financially important
- High volume
- High cost

Practical considerations
- Real problem
- Activity can be measured
- Standards can be set
- Adequate sample available
- Change can be effected
- Work worth the effort

Group support
- All enthusiastic about it
- Expertise available
- Effort required acceptable

lihood of remediable deficiencies in care. One study of hypertension in the community found evidence to support the rule of halves: *'that half of the hypertensive population is undetected, half of those detected are untreated, and in half of those treated hypertension is not controlled'* [39].

The key to assessing clinical importance was described by Williamson [1] as the concept of *'achievable health benefit not achieved'*. On this argument diabetes, which can be effectively managed, would be more highly rated than say, motor neurone disease, which although a serious condition, is not readily treatable.

Although secondary to improving quality of care, cost containment is an important concern of audit. High cost procedures are obvious candidates. A study of coronary angiography and coronary artery by-pass surgery found that 21% of the angiographies and 16% of the operations were inappropriate [40]. The authors recommended that the appropriateness of each potential operation be assessed *'to determine which patients should first be investigated and treated when resources are limited and waiting lists are long'*. Certain procedures, like grommet insertion, can also be of high cost because of their frequency. Assessing cost and more particularly the potential for savings is the province of health economics and there are several excellent textbooks on this subject [41, 42]. In view of the difficulties of estimating costs it may be necessary to consult a professional health economist.

Checking that a health care problem is real is an obvious step which is sometimes overlooked. For example one group decided to assess the appropriateness of referral of patients to physiotherapy, and mounted an audit to assess the extent of the problem. This subsequently revealed, as the physiotherapists were well aware, that all patients had been appropriately referred [2]. The unnecessary audit could have been avoided by checking first whether the problem was real. The practicality of a topic should also be assessed, considering each stage of the audit cycle in turn. The question to be asked is: can the project be completed with the existing resources in a reasonable time? The decision on what is practicable will depend on a balance between the available resources and the importance of the topic.

A visual method of evaluation

Presenting the evaluation of topics graphically can help resolve the priorities of topics for audit. One useful technique, modified from Seedhouse's rings of uncertainty [43], is to grade each topic on a scale of one (of little importance) to five (very important) on each of the four dimensions shown in Table 4.3. The scores can then be plotted on Figure 4.2, and the importance of a topic assessed from the extent the grades cluster near the centre of the diagram. Topics with all points plotted near the centre would be given a high priority, whereas those with two or more in the outer rings would in general be given a low priority. However a low rating on feasibility would lead immediately to a low overall rating, since there is little point in beginning an impractical study.

The technique can be illustrated by assessing an audit proposed by a consultant cardiologist who is concerned about the management of hypertension in a health authority. The condition can be well controlled and the consequences of not doing so are serious. As there is also evidence that it is poorly managed in up to 50% of cases [39], the topic scores highly on

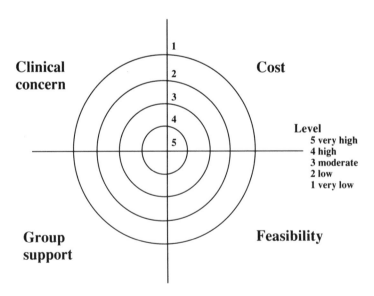

Figure 4.2   *Rings of evaluation*

clinical concern. Because of the high prevalence of hypertension it is financially important. Hypertension in the community also scores highly on all the practical considerations except whether change can be effected. Because it is largely managed in general practice, the cooperation of all the GPs in the health authority would be needed. Explaining the project to them, enlisting their support and encouraging them to change their practice presents many administrative and logistical difficulties. Thus the topic would attract a low score for practicability, and might well not be selected for audit. It is an example of a topic which would be ideal for one professional (a general practitioner), but inappropriate for another.

Refining a topic

When first identified topics may appear important but may be in a form which is not easy to audit, such as hypertension in the community. Some topics may need to be abandoned as impractical, but others can be modified to become more feasible. An example illustrates the principles.

The doctors who run an out-patient pain clinic are concerned to audit the quality of the care they give. They realise that the patients have such diverse problems and management that all cannot be covered in a single study. The doctors decide to select a particular group which is easily described and which is also one of the commonest problems that they see. The stated objective of the audit is: *to determine whether patients with low back pain are being effectively managed.*

Although this appears to be a focused study, it is vague. The topic has three components: the type of patient; the type of management; and the outcome of treatment. Each of these needs to be specified in more detail before a practical project can be designed. The term low back pain encompasses a variety of conditions for which different treatments are appropriate. Further there are different approaches to the management of patients whose pain problem is of recent onset and those who have been in pain for several years. The management of pain can involve physical treatments, such as drugs, surgery, electrical stimulation, nerve blocks or physiotherapy. A psychological approach might be adopted, developing coping strategies to enable the patient to manage despite the pain, or to deal with the adverse psychological effects that result from being in pain. It is clear that no single study could collect sufficient detail on all of these treatments to permit an assessment of the quality of care being given. Finally there is the problem of what is meant by effectiveness and how it can be measured. The objectives of pain management could be to improve: the control of pain; the control of the psychological consequences of pain; or the quality of life of the patient.

More specific questions lead directly to the design of the study of patients with low back pain:

- Are new patients given adequate instruction in the use of TENS (transcutaneous electrical nerve stimulation)?
- Were psychological assessments considered for patients who have had pain for more than two years?
- Were antidepressants tried early in the management of patients with nerve damage pain?

This example shows the aspects of the topic which were refined: the diagnostic group; the management; and the measures of success. Table 4.4 lists some of the points which could be considered; the exact list will depend on the particular topic.

Table 4.4   *Refining a topic*

Patient group
- Age
- Sex
- Diagnosis
- Disease duration
- Disease severity
- Referral source

Management
- Location of care
- Investigations
- Treatment
- Staff involved
- Duration of care

Outcome
- Cure
- Symptom control
- Time period

Refinement should produce a much simpler question with limited aims, which will clarify the data items which need to be collected, simplify decisions on the value and practicability of the audit, and simplify the setting of standards of care. Refining the topic can stimulate speculation about possible underlying causes of the supposed deficiency in health care and ways these might be remedied. In short, refining the topic should make it easier to improve the delivery of health care.

REVIEWING TOPICS COVERED

After an audit group has been operating for some time it is worth checking that the topics audited cover the range of areas of care. As experience in audit is gained, attention may become fixed on a few areas of health care to the exclusion of others. One way to identify whether this is happening is to review the types of patients, procedures and treatments which have been audited to see if any major groups have been omitted. The number of audits falling into the categories of structure, process, outcome and patient satisfaction could also be reviewed. This would show which types of audit predominate, and which areas of health care are relatively neglected. As part of this appraisal the audits could also be assessed to see which stage of the audit cycle was reached, in particular how many attempted to effect change and how many were successful. This will highlight those areas in which most progress is being made towards improving health care delivery, and identify those in which additional efforts are required. This type of assessment allows the audit group to review the progress it is making, and to make informed decisions so that the necessary actions can be taken.

SUMMARY

Topics for audit can be divided into:

- Structure—the health care facilities available.
- Process—the management given.
- Outcome—the result for the patient.
- Patient satisfaction.

Topics can be identified from a variety of sources, including:

- Literature review.
- Clinical experience.
- Case-note review.
- Surveys.

There are many potential topics, and selection for further study should depend on:

- Clinical importance.
- Cost.
- Feasibility.
- Enthusiasm of the audit group.

When first suggested, topics may be phrased in general terms, in a form which makes study design difficult. The topic may need to be refined. As successive audits are undertaken, the types of topics being studied should be reviewed to ensure that important areas for audit are not being overlooked.

REFERENCES

1. Williamson JW. Formulating priorities for quality assurance activity. J Am Med Assoc 1978; 239: 631–7.
2. Baker R. Problem solving with audit in general practice. Br Med J 1990; 300: 378–80.
3. Thin RNT. Workloads in genitourinary medicine clinics in England. Genitourin Med 1989; 65: 376–81.
4. Elkind A, Eardley A, Thompson R, Smith A. How district health authorities organise cervical screening. Br Med J 1990; 301: 915–8.
5. Haiart DC, Paul AB, Griffiths JMT. An audit of the usage of operating theatre time in a peripheral teaching surgical unit. Postgrad Med J 1990; 66: 612–5.
6. Fisher RB, Dearden CH. Improving the care of patients with major trauma in the accident and emergency department. Br Med J 1990; 300: 1560–3.
7. Adler MW. A unique opportunity to upgrade genitourinary medicine. Br Med J 1989; 298: 1201–2.

8. Marber M, MacRae C, Joy M. Delay to invasive investigation and revascularisation for coronary heart disease in South West Thames region: a two tier system? Br Med J 1991; 302: 1189–91.

9. Beeley L. Safer prescribing. London: Blackwell, 1992.

10. Morgan DJR, Sutters CA, Pugh S. Medical audit and formulary management: a policy for rational use of thrombolytic drugs. Postgrad Med J 1991; 67: 165–9.

11. Roberts CJ. Annotation: towards the more effective use of diagnostic radiology: a review of the work of the Royal College of Radiologists' working party on the more effective use of diagnostic radiology, 1976 to 1988. Clin Radiol 1988; 39: 3–6.

12. Samanta A, Haider Y, Roffe C. An audit of patients attending a general medical follow-up clinic. J R Coll Physicians London 1991; 25: 33–5.

13. O'Dwyer FG, D'Alton A, Pearce JB. Adolescent self harm patients: audit of assessment in an accident and emergency department. Br Med J 1991; 303: 629–30.

14. Whitty P, Parker C, Prieto-Ramos F, Al-Kharusi S. Communication of results of necropsies in North East Thames region. Br Med J 1991; 303: 1244–6.

15. Epstein AM. The outcomes movement—will it get us where we want to go? N Engl J Med 1990; 323: 266–9.

16. Godber G. The confidential enquiry into maternal deaths. In: McLachlan G, ed. A Question of Quality. London: Oxford University Press, 1976: 24–33.

17. Campling EA, Devlin HB, Lunn JN. The report of the national confidential enquiry into perioperative deaths 1989. London: Disc to Print Ltd, 1990.

18. Rutstein DD, Berenberg W, Chalmers TC, Child CG, Fishman AP, Perrin EB. Measuring the quality of medical care: a clinical method. N Engl J Med 1976; 294: 582–8.

19. Scott DL, Haslock I. Measuring performance in clinical rheumatology. Ann Rheum Dis 1990; 49: 3–5.

20. Cappell HM, Cox N, Dawes P, Dieppe P, Geney J, Griffiths I, et al. Guidelines for audit measures for specialist supervision of patients with rheumatoid arthritis. J R Coll Physicians London 1992; 26: 76–82.

21. Kemple TJ, Hayter SR. Audit of diabetes in general practice. Br Med J 1991; 302: 451–3.

22. Fries JF. Towards an understanding of patient outcome measurement. Arthritis Rheum 1983; 26: 697–704.

23. Gore SM, Taylor RMR, Wallwork J. Availability of transplantable organs from brain stem dead donors in intensive care units. Br Med J 1991; 302: 149–53.

24.   Nobrega FT, Morrow GW, Smoldt RK, Offord KP. Quality assessment in hypertension: analysis of process and outcome methods. N Engl J Med 1977; 296: 145–8.
25.   Munday PE. Genitourninary medicine services; consumers' views. Genitourin Med 1991; 66: 108–11.
26.   Schofield MJ, Bennet A, Redman S, Walters WAW, Sanson-Fisher RW. Self-reported long-term outcomes of hysterectomy. Br J Obstet Gynaecol 1991; 98: 1129–36.
27.   Hopkins A, Maxwell R. Contracts and quality of care. Br Med J 1990; 300: 919–22.
28.   Fitzpatrick R. Survey of patient satisfaction: I—Important general considerations. Br Med J 1991; 302: 887–9.
29.   Doyle BJ, Ware JE. Physician conduct and other factors that affect consumer satisfaction with medical care. J Med Educ 1977; 52: 793–801.
30.   Hall JA, Dorman MC. What patients like about their medical care and how often they are asked: a meta-analysis of the satisfaction literature. Soc Sci Med 1988; 27: 935–9.
31.   Fitzpatrick R. Surveys of patient satisfaction: II—Designing a questionnaire and conducting a survey. Br Med J 1991; 302: 1129–32.
32.   Shaw CD. Aspects of Audit: 5. Looking forward to audit. Br Med J 1980; i: 1509–11.
33.   Difford F. Defining essential data for audit in general practice. Br Med J 1990; 300: 92–4.
34.   Royal College of Obstetricians and Gynaecologists. Second Bulletin. Medical Audit Unit, 1991.
35.   Joint Working Party of the Royal College of Pathologists, the Royal College of Physicians of London, and the Royal College of Surgeons of England. The autopsy and audit. London: RCPath, RCP, RCS, 1991.
36.   Irvin TT. Abdominal pain: a surgical audit of 1190 emergency admissions. Br J Surg 1989; 76: 1121–5.
37.   UK-TIA Study Group. Variation in the use of angiography and carotid endarterectomy by neurologists in the UK-TIA aspirin trial. Br Med J 1983; 286: 514–7.
38.   Gruer R, Gordon DS, Gunn AA, Ruckley CV. Audit of surgical audit. Lancet 1986; i: 23–6.
39.   Smith WCS, Lee AJ, Crombie IK, Tunstall-Pedoe H. Control of blood pressure in Scotland: the rule of halves. Br Med J 1990; 300: 981–3.
40.   Gray D, Hampton JR, Bernstein SJ, Kosecoff J, Brook RH. Audit of coronary angiography and bypass surgery. Lancet 1990; 335: 1317–20.

41. Drummond MF. Principles of economic appraisal in health care. Oxford: Oxford University Press, 1990.
42. Mooney GH. Economics, medicine and health care. London: Harvester Wheatsheaf, 1986.
43. Seedhouse D. Liberating medicine. London: Wiley, 1990.

5

Standards

The use of defined standards of medical care is the hallmark of audit. Standards are a formal statement of how well patients should be managed, with the understanding that this level of care should be as high as resources allow. Their primary purpose is to highlight deficiencies, by clarifying the care which should be given. When care is manifestly poor, as Florence Nightingale found in 19th Century Crimea (see Chapter 1), standards may not be needed. Today deficiencies in care are often subtle and some means of identifying them is needed. Standards fill this role.

The value of a standard for audit depends crucially on the way it is framed. A possible standard for the management of hypertension could be adequate control of blood pressure. This is too general, for it leaves unspecified what level of blood pressure is adequate and it takes no account of possible exceptions, like refractory hypertension associated with renal disease. The setting of specific, realistic standards of care, which are acceptable to all those involved, is a major challenge for audit. This chapter reviews the nature of standards and the problems of setting them.

THE NATURE OF STANDARDS

Standards are usually represented as a single stage of the audit cycle, but they fill three separate roles:

- Foster discussion.
- Highlight problems.
- Motivate change.

Developing standards helps to focus attention on a health care problem, fostering discussion among colleagues and reading of relevant literature. This helps fulfil the educational aim of audit. Comparing standards against current practice can confirm the existence of the problems which might otherwise have remained hidden. Finally, by illuminating the gulf between current practice and the desired level of care, the standard may help motivate change. When an audit group has agreed that a certain level of care should be provided, finding that current practice falls below this can act as a spur to action.

A well known example of a standard is one which the government has set for general practice; 80% of eligible women should be screened for cervical cancer for the general practitioner to receive the higher level of payment [1]. This illustrates two facets of standards: the criterion; and the target attained. In this case the criterion is whether cervical screening was carried out; and the target is that 80% of women should meet the criterion. The standard could be extended by adding the proviso, the allowable exception, that those who are not at risk of cervical cancer could be excluded from the calculation of the target. Allowable exceptions can be important; when the target for cervical cytology was set *'the profession expressed grave concerns about the ethics of introducing pressures on general practitioners to undertake procedures in doubtful clinical circumstances'* [1].

Criteria

Criteria are based on clinical observations or measurements which assess the quality of care a patient has received. For many conditions a criterion will define an acceptable level of a physiological measure: blood sugar of <10 mmol/l for insulin dependent diabetes; diastolic blood pressure of <90 mmHg for hypertensive patients. For other conditions it may involve recording whether an event occurred: administration of thrombolytic drugs within six hours of a myocardial infarction; the occurrence of rebleeding in gastrointestinal haemorrhage. Criteria are not meant to provide a summary of all aspects of care, but to focus attention on key items which are indicative of good care. This leads to the three requirements of good criteria. They should be:

- Clinically relevant.
- Clearly defined.
- Easily measured.

The four examples given above easily fulfil these requirements. They are clinically relevant because they are important for good management. The less important the criterion is to good outcome the less valuable it is. Poorly chosen criteria can even lead to adequate care being falsely classed as inadequate; in one extreme instance, when poor general criteria were used, 95% of well managed cases were falsely classed as inadequate [2]. Good criteria need to focus on critical aspects of care. The methods for identifying and refining topics (Chapter 4) can also be used to derive good criteria.

The need for clearly defined and easily measured criteria is evident. Sometimes this is straightforward: all-or-none criteria such as post-operative death or nosocomial infection satisfy both requirements. Many of the outcome measures listed in Chapter 4 could be used as all-or-none criteria. Physiological values, such as proteinuria in pregnancy or peak flow in asthma, are easily measured, but the definition of the criterion requires a little thought. A cut-off level which distinguishes between good and inadequate care needs to be set. For many routine measurements the cut-off value will be well known.

Some types of criteria present problems both for definition and measurement. For example, quality of life in rheumatoid arthritis or cognitive function following stroke are both attractive subjects for criteria, but they present problems. How can quality of life be measured? and what level of quality of life indicates good care? Methods of measuring these outcomes are reviewed in Chapter 7.

Implicit criteria

The examples of criteria given above, involving physical measurements or defined observations, are referred to as objective or explicit. Assessing whether or not a death during an asthma attack was preventable is a different kind of observation from making a physical measurement. It represents a second type of criterion, described as subjective or implicit because it uses clinical judgement to assess the quality of care. In many instances decisions on care will require clinical judgement, for example whether investigations or treatments were appropriate, or whether the time to diagnosis or the length of hospital stay were unnecessarily prolonged. An audit of patients in an acute psychiatric rehabilitation unit used a multidisciplinary team to assess the appropriateness of discharge [3]. It found that almost half the bed days were occupied by patients ready to be discharged, but who could not be found adequate accommodation.

One advantage of clinical judgement is its flexibility; a series of patients with different types of problem can be assessed. The limitation of subjective measures is that important deficiencies in care can be overlooked. A common finding with subjective measures is that different observers may come to different conclusions. One study in general medicine found that when clinicians reassessed the quality of care they changed their minds in 16% of cases [4]. When objective measures can be used they are, in general, to be preferred.

Use of management guidelines

One way to strengthen subjective criteria is to employ a management plan in the form of a clinical algorithm. An audit of the management of acute asthma used guidelines similar to those produced by the British Thoracic Society to assess 76 adults admitted to hospital [5]. The guidelines enabled a number of deficiencies in immediate and long term management to be identified, and there was a high level of agreement between the assessments given by different observers. There are now many sets of guidelines covering a range of conditions, often issued under the auspices of the Royal Colleges [6]. Establishing such guidelines is a complex time-consuming task, and although potentially rewarding, is beyond the scope of most audit groups.

Guidelines and clinical algorithms, although useful, should be used with some care in audit. There may be a temptation to collect data on each component of what is considered good management. For some guidelines this would involve a great many items and in any given patient many of the components will not be relevant. The result would be to increase the cost of data collection and make the analysis more complicated. Some groups in the United States have prepared comprehensive lists of criteria for selected conditions. One, for diabetes, contains 133 items covering all possible diagnostic information and all possible management programmes [7]. To enable the list to be used the criteria are arranged as a branching flow chart so that only a few are relevant to any given patient. The resulting *'criteria map'* is large and would require some training before it could be used. This approach seems more suited to an overall assessment of quality than one intended to identify and resolve health care problems. There is much to commend the alternative view of *'keep it short, keep it simple'*.

Key items which distinguish between good and poor care can be selected from the guidelines, simplifying data collection and interpretation. If data on many items are collected, departures from some of the minor ones may, for individual patients, be clinically defensible, leading to arguments about what kind of departures constitute poor care. Guidelines can point towards good criteria, but by themselves they are not standards. Because they are primarily an aid to good management, their main role in audit is as a means of improving care (see Chapter 8).

Targets

The target to be attained is the proportion of the patients seen who should meet the criterion. For cervical screening this was 80% of eligible women. For adverse outcomes, such as postoperative wound infection, the target will be set low, perhaps close to zero. For other processes, such as the administration of anti-D immunoglobulin to rhesus negative women who have had a rhesus positive baby, the target would be high, close to 100%. The level at which the target is set is a compromise between three factors:

- Clinical importance.
- Practicability.
- Acceptability.

Although it would be preferable for all patients to receive the highest standards of care, in practice this may not be possible. Some patients will not comply with drug treatment, or the results of investigations may be delayed or even incorrect. The level at which the target is set will depend on the balance between practicability and importance.

The target must also be one that all participants think is attainable. If an ambitious target were not met in an audit study, there is a danger that evidence of a health care problem would be rejected because the target level was too high. To overcome this, the idea of minimum and optimum targets has been introduced [8]. A minimum target corresponds to *'the least we can do'*, whereas an optimum target is what, on balance, *'we think we ought to achieve'*. It might be possible to reach a higher target, an ideal, but the time and effort which this would require is not justified. To do so would consume resources which could be spent more effectively in other ways. For example the uptake of cervical screening in general practice could be raised by discussing with non-attenders the benefits of screening and trying to allay any doubts or fears they may have. However this one-to-one counselling would be very time-consuming, and might only achieve a small increase in uptake. The time spent would be at the expense of other activities like screening for cardiovascular risk factors, or increasing the uptake of childhood immunisation. Thus targets have to be set in the context of clinical work, where all involved agree that the effort of attaining the target is justified by the expected improvements in health care.

Once the target has been set, the criterion must be measured on a large enough group of patients to get a clear picture of the level of care being given. For example, consider a cardiology clinic which set the target that 80% of hypertensive patients should be adequately controlled. If it had achieved this target, would a sample of 20 hypertensives be large enough to show this? The answer is probably not. Because of the play of chance there is a probability of 60% that the sample value would be lower than the target, even if among all hypertensives being seen in the clinic 80% were adequately controlled. This calculation uses a simple statistical procedure (the binomial distribution), and although the details of it do not concern us the implications do. Small samples can give misleading estimates of the quality of medical care. On the other hand, unnecessarily large ones waste resources. The question of how big samples need to be is addressed in more detail in Chapter 6.

Unstated targets

Many, indeed most, published audit studies do not state a target, but simply interpret their findings as indicating good or poor care. Sometimes this does not matter as the implication of the findings is clear. An audit of the management of myocardial infarction found that 74% of eligible patients received thrombolytic therapy [9]. The authors decided this was unacceptably low, and instituted changes which increased it to 91%.

Unfortunately in the absence of stated targets there is a danger that the audit findings may be interpreted as a vindication of current practice. Current practice may indeed be good, but the aim of audit is to improve it. An audit of amniocentesis in a district general hospital illustrates this problem. It described several features of the process of care and of outcome, but concluded only that complication rates were acceptable, and recommended that the audit should not be repeated [10]. Perhaps more extreme is an audit of asthma which found that 16 out of 35 deaths were potentially preventable but concluded '*nevertheless, most of the hospital deaths (19/35) were considered not to have been preventable*' [11]. These authors were highly critical of many aspects of care, but in their assessment of avoidable mortality seemed to imply that better than 50% is somehow acceptable.

Allowable exceptions

There will be circumstances in which criteria do not apply to certain patients. For example cervical screening would not be appropriate for women who have had cervicectomies. Specifying allowable exceptions enables cases to be removed from the audit, simplifying the comparison of the target with current practice. It might be possible to allow for these exceptions by lowering the target level, but this would require that the frequency of allowable exceptions be known accurately. Removing them from the audit also prevents arguments of the kind *'I didn't meet the target because some of my cases were special'*.

One common type of allowable exception is concurrent illness, but social and personal factors can also be important. For example, home circumstances can determine whether an early discharge is possible, or whether in-patient care would have to be extended until a place in a nursing home could be found. A study of admissions to a provincial hospital found that 10% of bed days were inappropriate because social reasons prevented discharge [12].

TYPES OF STANDARDS

Standards are sometimes recommended by prestigious organisations, but are often decided by the audit group itself. The distinction leads to two types of standard: external and internal.

External

External standards are set by bodies such as the Government or the Royal Colleges, and are imposed on individual practitioners. The most comprehensive set of external targets are those published by the World Health Organisation as part of its Health For All By The Year 2000 [13]. In total 38 targets were set for the European region, covering specific diseases, lifestyles, the environment, and health care systems. Many of the targets were ideal, being goals to aim at rather than realistic objectives, for example, Target 5: 'by the year 2000, there will be no indigenous measles, poliomyelitis, neonatal tetanus, congenital rubella, diphtheria, congenital syphilis, or indigenous malaria in the region'. In contrast target 10 is more realistic: 'by the year 2000, mortality in the region from cancer among people under 65 should be reduced by at least 15%'. The proposed change is more modest, and the suggested solutions, reduction in smoking and improved cervical screening, should have some effect even if the target is not met. The timescale for achieving these targets is now recognised to have been too ambitious, and the phrase 'by the year 2000' has been deleted.

Sometimes guidelines are issued in place of fixed standards, in the hope that compliance with the guidelines will move practice towards some unstated target. Concern that current practice of caesarean section in Canada 'was not congruent with available research evidence' led to a national consensus conference which issued guidelines on the indications for caesarean section [14]. Unfortunately, despite widespread dissemination, the guidelines failed to promote the desired change (see Chapter 8).

Internal

Internal standards are negotiated within the audit group, with discussion leading to decisions on the criterion, the target and the allowable exceptions. The differences between internal and external standards are summarised in Table 5.1. The main advantage of internal standards is the sense of ownership which they endow: 'doctors who have created their own standards will be motivated to implement the product of their own work' [8]. In contrast externally set standards may be resented. However ownership is not without cost; time is needed to obtain information on which to base discussions and to achieve consensus on a desirable, attainable target. Because of this it has been suggested that internal standards may, in some instances, be based on inadequate information. In contrast, external standards, particularly those emanating from the colleges or consensus conferences, may have a higher degree of rigour. One solution is to take external standards where they are available and modify them to take account of local circumstances.

Table 5.1   *Comparison of external and internal standards*

External	Internal
Imposed	Negotiated
Remote	Sense of ownership
Usually authoritative	Sometimes non-rigorous
Fixed	Adaptable to local circumstances
No effort for local group	Considerable effort
Disincentive to further improvement	Evolve to maximum worthwhile

Internal standards can be set at the level that the audit group think realistic. Again the benefit is not without cost; the group may be tempted to set a lower standard to ensure that it is reached. This is not necessarily a serious problem if standards are not immutable, but are recognised as evolving.

Evolving standards

The evolution of standards is a feature of good audit, because the audit cycle can be negotiated more than once (see Chapter 2). After the first pass through the cycle the standard would be re-assessed, asking *'how much additional improvement can be achieved at reasonable cost?'*. In an audit of wound infection following colorectal surgery the percentage of infected wounds was progressively lowered from 43% to 31% to 18% to 1% [15]. Although each step represented a major improvement, additional changes to the antibiotic treatment were easy to implement so that changes were made until a very high standard was reached.

This form of evolving standards meets one of the criticisms sometimes raised against standards, that a fixed target will discourage attempts to improve beyond it. A commonly cited example of this is the government target for childhood immunisation in general practice; once the figure of 90% is reached there will be no incentive to improve beyond it. But, if the audit group has agreed that a topic is important then it will want to assess the magnitude of the remaining health care problem at the end of each audit so that an informed decision can be taken whether further improvement is warranted.

SETTING STANDARDS

Setting standards is a convenient phrase and widely used (including in this book), but in some ways it is an unfortunate one. It carries a sense of imposition, which is only appropriate for external standards prescribed by an outside body. The essence of internal standards is that all participants agree that an important aspect of care is being measured, and the target is one which should be reached. Decisions will usually be made through a combination of clinical experience and a review of the available evidence, but will only be arrived at after discussion with all involved. Reaching agreement raises the issues of decision-making in groups which were reviewed in Chapter 3.

Whether internal or external standards are used, good information is essential to their formation. One study in Canada found that a panel of 10 gave similar assessments in 85% of cases when good research evidence was available, but did so in only 30% of cases when the evidence was poor or conflicting [16]. Evidence can be obtained from several sources:

- Literature review.
- Comparison with other centres.
- Clinical judgement.
- Assessment of current practice.

Literature review

The best sources are the published reports from other centres, particularly acknowledged centres of excellence. To be as good as the best is a simple standard to set, and one likely to appeal to many. Standards can also be obtained from national guidelines or from the statements from the Royal Colleges. However, when these sources are used, it is important that the standards are discussed by the audit group to ensure that all are in agreement. Local circumstances, such as non-availability of expensive diagnostic facilities, may mean the target is not attainable and a lower one should be set.

Comparison with other centres

Comparisons with other centres or regions can reveal possible shortcomings in care. When audit is being carried out at regional level, it may be possible to use official health care statistics. For example Charlton and colleagues [17] compared mortality rates in the 98 area health authorities in England and Wales. They focused on conditions which are amenable to medical intervention and found substantial variation in death rates from diseases which *'should be largely avoidable by efficient and effective health care'*. However in many instances the data required to make comparisons between centres will not be available from official sources and special surveys will need to be conducted. This was the approach which the Royal College of Radiologists adopted to set a standard for preoperative chest X-rays (POCR). It found that the frequency of these investigations between centres ranged from 11.5% to 54.2%. It argued that *'in view of the absence of clinical usefulness of routine POCR ... there is a case for setting a temporary norm for POCR in non-acute, non-cardiopulmonary surgery at the lowest level of utilisation found in the eight centres (12%)'* [18]. Another group studied the management of chronic pain in out-patients [19] and found large differences in the patterns of referral of patients to the clinics and in their management. Surveys can provide many interesting findings but their role is limited. They are easy to do if the centres already have routine data collection systems in place, otherwise they are expensive. Interpreting the findings also presents problems. The likelihood is that there will be differences in types of patients seen at each of the centres, so that different approaches to management may be justified. This issue, of the interpretation of the findings of audit studies, is reviewed in Chapter 9.

Clinical judgement

Often there will be no information on which to base a target, placing reliance on clinical judgement, on a best guess, of what level of care should be achieved. When *process* is being assessed, setting targets in this way may sometimes not be too difficult.

For example with stroke patients a rough estimate could be made of the proportion who should have a CT scan, or the proportion for whom definite diagnosis should be made within three days. Setting targets may also be possible for certain unexpected adverse events: again for stroke patients a guess could be made of the proportion who might suffer bed sores, or develop respiratory infection. In contrast guessing *outcome* is different: specifying how many stroke patients should recover full independence at three months, or how many will need no assistance with eating, is more difficult. Targets which are set in these circumstances will often be arbitrary and may be challenged because of this.

Assessment of current practice

Direct observation of the way care is being delivered can also be used to set standards. Many audits begin with a brief assessment of current practice to determine whether there is a deficiency in care. The preliminary findings may also stimulate the interest of the group. Clinical judgement is used to decide whether improvements need to be made; the question asked is *'are we doing as well as we think we should?'*. Sometimes the answer is obvious. When a review of patients attending a genitourinary clinic revealed that *'only about a quarter of homosexual and bisexual men presenting as new patients ... and assumed to be susceptible to hepatitis B virus infection were effectively immunised'*, the auditors immediately recognised the problem and titled their report: *'Failure to deliver hepatitis B vaccine: confessions from a genitourinary medicine clinic'* [20]. However, in some instances, when explicit standards are not available, the interpretation of the findings can be problematic. Reporting an audit of the appropriateness of hospital referral for hypertension the authors stated that it was not possible to set a standard because, *'we do not know, however what is an acceptable proportion of inappropriate referrals'* [21]. When they found that almost 60% of referrals failed to meet the primary criterion of appropriateness, the authors were unable to draw conclusions, and did not suggest whether improvement was needed. This difficulty is likely to arise when the aim of the audit is simply to monitor current practice, rather than discover whether and to what extent the delivery of care could be improved. When the audit group is committed to improving care instead of merely observing it, the difficulties of setting standards will be lessened. At the end of each audit the concern will be less with whether an arbitrary standard was met, than with how much additional improvement could be achieved.

SUMMARY

The term standards is used in a particular way in audit. Standards play an essential role, but setting them is one the most difficult stages of audit.

- *Uses of standards*
  Standards in audit have three components, the criterion, the target and the allowable exceptions. The primary use of standards is to highlight deficiencies in care. Standards can also stimulate discussion of particular health care problems.
- *Criterion*
  The criterion states the specific aspect of care which should be achieved. If the criterion is not formally stated, deficiencies in care may be overlooked.
- *Target*
  The target is the proportion of patients in whom the criterion should be met. The target should be stated before the audit is undertaken. Unstated targets can lead to a vindication of present practice, whether it be good or bad. The target should be realistic and all members of the audit group should agree that it is attainable and worthwhile.
- *Allowable exceptions*
  There may be patients to whom, for medical or social reasons, the criterion does not apply. These allowable exceptions are excluded from the calculation of targets.
- *Guidelines*
  Guidelines for patient management are different from standards used in audit. Guidelines describe all the salient features of patient management, whereas standards focus on selected aspects of management, specifying the target to be attained. Inspection of guidelines can suggest criteria.

- *External standards*
  Standards of care are sometimes set by external bodies such as the government, Royal Colleges, or consensus conferences. These may be resisted, a common argument being that they are unrealistic given local circumstances. They do however indicate optimal levels of care which could be achieved.
- *Internal standards*
  Internal standards, negotiated within the audit group, are more likely to encourage adherence than external ones. They can be developed from external ones by group discussion, when local circumstances can be taken into account.
- *Evolving standards*
  Standards are not immutable. They evolve over successive audits towards improved levels of care. The aim of the auditors is to improve health care as far as is practical.
- *Negotiating standards*
  Standards can be agreed following literature review, comparison of performance against other centres, or by critical assessment of current practice. All relevant staff should be involved in discussions so that the standard is one which all want to achieve, rather than one imposed by others.

REFERENCES

1. Chisholm JW. The 1990 contract: its history and its content. Br Med J 1990; 300: 853–6.
2. Sanazaro PJ, Mills DH. A critique of the use of generic screening in quality assessment. J Am Med Assoc 1991; 265: 1977–81.
3. Dick PH, Crombie IK, Durham T, McFee C, Primrose M, Mitchell S. Unnecessary hospitalisation in a psychiatric rehabilitation unit. Br Med J 1992; 304: 1544.
4. Brook RH, Appel FA. Quality-of-care assessment: choosing a method for peer review. N Engl J Med 1973; 288: 1323–9.
5. Bell D, Layton AJ, Gabbay J. Use of a guideline based questionnaire to audit hospital care of acute asthma. Br Med J 1991; 302: 1440–3.
6. Jenkins D. Investigations: how to get from guidelines to protocols. Br Med J 1991; 303: 323–4.
7. Greenfield S, Lewis CE, Kaplan SH, Davidson MB. Peer review by criteria mapping: criteria for diabetes mellitus. Ann Intern Med 1975; 83: 761–70.

8. Irvine D, Irvine S. Making sense of audit. Oxford: Radcliffe Medical Press, 1991.

9. Lewis F, Jishi F, Sissons CE, Baker JT, Child DF. Value of emergency cardiac enzymes: audit in a coronary care unit. J R Soc Med 1991; 84: 398-9.

10. Wiener JJ, Farrow A, Farrow SC. Audit of amniocentesis from a district health centre: is it worth it? Br Med J 1990; 300: 1243-5.

11. Eason J, Markowe HLJ. Controlled investigation of deaths from asthma in hospitals in the North East Thames region. Br Med J 1987; 294: 1255-8.

12. Anderson P, Meara J, Brodhurst S, Attwood S, Timbrell M, Gatherer A. Use of hospital beds: a cohort study of admissions to a provincial teaching hospital. Br Med J 1988; 297: 910-12.

13. World Health Organisation. Targets for Health For All. Copenhagen: WHO, 1985.

14. Lomas J, Anderson GM, Domnick-Pierre K, Vayda E, Enkin MW, Hannah WJ. Do practice guidelines guide practice? The effect of a consensus statement on the practice of physicians. N Engl J Med 1989; 321: 1306-11.

15. Hancock BD. Audit of major colorectal and biliary surgery to reduce rates of wound infection. Br Med J 1990; 301: 911-12.

16. Lomas J, Anderson G, Enkind M, Vayda E, Roberts R, Mackinnon B. The role of evidence in the consensus process. J Am Med Assoc 1988; 259: 3001-5.

17. Charlton JRH, Hartley RM, Silver R, Holland WW. Geographical variation in mortality from conditions amenable to medical intervention in England and Wales. Lancet 1983; i: 691-6.

18. National Study by The Royal College of Radiologists. Preoperative chest radiology. Lancet 1979; ii: 83-6.

19. Crombie IK, Davies HTO. Audit in outpatients: entering the loop. Br Med J 1991; 302: 1437-9.

20. Bhatti N, Gilson RJC, Beecham M, Williams P, Matthews MP, Tedder RS, et al. Failure to deliver hepatitis B vaccine: confessions from a genitourinary medicine clinic. Br Med J 1991; 303: 97-101.

21. Juncosa S, Jones RB, McGhee SM. Appropriateness of hospital referral for hypertension. Br Med J 1990; 300: 646-8.

6

Methods of Audit

Methods of audit range in sophistication and complexity from single case presentations to multi-centre surveys involving computer analysis of data collected on thousands of patients. The diversity reflects the variety of topics for audit, each method being suited to certain types of topic. There is no single best method of audit. This chapter describes the methods in detail, showing how they are used and outlining their advantages and limitations.

Strictly speaking these are not *methods* of audit. A true method of audit would cover all the stages of the audit cycle, reviewed in Chapter 2, from selecting a topic through to effecting change. Instead, *methods of audit* are simply different ways of carrying out part of the audit cycle, the collection of data on current practice. In this text we follow convention and refer to them as methods of audit, while recognising that the practice of audit involves much more than data collection.

Data collection holds a strange fascination, so that it is often begun before a study is properly planned (see Chapter 10). Many audit projects, because they focus primarily on the acquisition of data, do not use their findings to improve health care. Data may lead to information and thence to understanding, but unless used in a planned programme, they will contribute little towards improving the delivery of care. Thus to clarify the role of methods, this chapter also reviews the purposes served by audit data.

CASE-NOTE BASED STUDIES

Case-notes are the most obvious sources of data, and have been used for various methods of audit:

- Case presentation.
- Adverse events.
- Occurrence screening.
- Criterion based audit.

The different approaches vary primarily in the number and type of patients audited.

Case presentation/review

The simplest form of audit involves reviewing the management of individual cases. This is not the conventional case presentation in which cases are selected because they illustrate interesting or unusual clinical features: *'the usual clinical meeting, or "grand round", while desirable, is not sufficient for the requirements of clinical audit because of the non-random selection of patients, a bias towards unusual medical conditions and, often, the lack of attention to administrative and communication matters'* [1]. The key features of the case review method are summarised in Table 6.1. A common format is for meetings of up to one hour to be held once a fortnight [2]. The key to successful meetings is to ensure that they take place in *'a friendly, non-confrontational manner'* [3]. In practice the recommendation that *'the essential nature of audit is a frank discussion between doctors, on a regular basis and without fear of criticism'* [4], may be difficult to achieve. One way to overcome the natural reluctance of health professionals to discuss shortcomings in patient management is for senior staff to volunteer some of their own cases for early review. For example Heath [3] reported an audit presentation, concerning a patient of his who *'was prescribed spironolactone at a time when the serum potassium concentration was >6 mmol/l'*.

Table 6.1   *Key points about case presentation*

Meetings
- friendly, non-confrontational
- weekly or fortnightly
- one hour

Decisions
- which cases?
- who reviews them?
- which assessment method?

Advantages
- simple
- cheap
- quick

Disadvantages
- small number of cases
- usually subjective assessments
- possibly threatening

The broader implications of the finding for clinical practice were discussed at an audit meeting and ward practice was modified to ensure that investigations were taken into account when prescribing. Other strategies to overcome anxiety were reviewed in Chapter 3.

Case presentation requires careful preparation, the first question being which cases to review. One group, set up in Birmingham in 1978, randomly selected cases from all those seen [3]. This approach had some success, particularly the improvement of the quality of case-notes, but became somewhat repetitive [5]. Doubts about the usefulness of random selection of cases were also expressed by a group from London who found 'dissatisfactions' and 'alienation' following repeated general audits [6]. They also reported that audits which focused on specific topics, such as management of pulmonary embolus or gastrointestinal bleeding, were much more popular, prompted vigorous discussion, and were thought to be educationally valuable.

The quality of care which was given can be assessed in different ways. Deficiencies in management can be identified using clinical judgement while reviewing the notes. Alternatively a checklist of points, such as the appropriateness of investigations and treatments, or the timeliness and quality of contact with other clinicians involved, can be used in the review.

Although clinical judgement is more flexible, and can cover a wider range of items than a simple checklist, it has the disadvantage of being subjective (see Chapter 5).

The main advantage of case presentation is its simplicity, involving little administrative time and without need for computers or statistical analysis. This simplicity means that it is always worth considering first when planning an audit. Audit groups can mount this type of audit and, if it is successful, see the benefits very quickly. A limitation of this method is that only a small number of cases can be reviewed so that some major deficiencies in health care may not be audited.

Adverse events

Rather than focusing on particular conditions, cases may be selected because they are likely to contain serious, clear cut, management errors. For example cases of unplanned return to an operating theatre or unexpected death would be expected to contain more instances of sub-optimal care than randomly selected cases. In the United States this has been described as focusing on the *'airplane crashes in health'* [7]. This practice is well established in Britain in the form of the surgical morbidity and mortality meetings which, following College recommendations, should be held at every hospital [2]. Each case is assessed by the surgical team to determine whether there were deficiencies in care and, if so, to identify reasons for them.

Adverse events are surprisingly common; experience in Britain suggests that they occur in about 20% of patients, in keeping with American findings [8]. The most common are hospital acquired infections, but cardiac and respiratory arrest and accidental falls are also prominent. A list of adverse events which could be used for this type of audit was presented in Chapter 4. This method, being a variant on case presentation, has the same advantages and limitations, except that objective criteria for the assessment of adverse events can be employed.

Occurrence screening

The audit of adverse events can be extended so that instead of assessing one or two cases, a series of patients is reviewed.

This technique, which again is widely used in the United States, is known as occurrence screening [8]. Trained staff, usually qualified nurses, screen the cases using a set of criteria which specify departures from good quality care. The criteria may be general and be applicable to all types of patients, such as the occurrence of bed sores or nosocomial infection. Alternatively they may be specific to certain conditions or types of patients, such as low apgar scores or failure to aspirate synovial fluid in patients with acute hot joint. Cases in which putative adverse events have occurred are peer reviewed and may be presented at audit meetings. The findings on all cases are collated to identify patterns in the data, simplifying the task of identifying the underlying reasons for deficiencies in the quality of care (see Chapter 8).

Criterion based audit

The emphasis of occurrence screening is on serious, clear cut adverse events. In many instances patients may have received sub-optimal care, recovering more slowly or only partially, without having experienced an obvious adverse event. Criterion based audit addresses this limitation by using a trained non-clinical reviewer to review all instances of sub-optimal care, whether or not they result in an adverse event [9].

In criterion based audit, a set of criteria specifying good management is developed during discussions among clinicians. The success of these methods depends on keeping the list of criteria short and simple to apply. Shaw [9] recommends: *'a limited number (12–15) of simple questions that can be answered yes or no'*. This focuses the audit onto *'key elements in management'* rather than specifying a complete protocol for clinical management. Guidelines prepared by the Royal Colleges and others provide a useful starting point in selecting criteria. Clinical experience and good judgement are then needed to select the key elements from these sometimes lengthy guidelines. The criteria used in criterion based audit are similar to those used in setting standards (see Chapter 5). The same methods can be employed to assess and identify clear and focused criteria.

Carefully designed, criterion based audit may provide one of the most efficient methods of audit. Its characteristics, simplicity and the use of trained non-clinical staff for data gathering should enable many topics to be audited. Even the detailed planning required for the development of criteria can be beneficial, focusing attention on the topic and increasing the sense of ownership of the audit among the clinicians involved. Because the method is comparatively recent its success in this country is not yet proven. Like all the case-note based methods, it depends on the availability and quality of case-notes.

Limitations of case-notes

Case-notes are clearly an excellent source of data for audit, but they have limitations:

- Availability.
- Completeness and quality of data.
- Identification of particular patients.

Case-notes are not always available for assessment; in some studies only one third of the relevant notes were located [10, 11]. The non-availability of notes is a problem because of the potential bias which it can introduce. Notes are more likely to be missing when patients are attending other clinics, have been readmitted to hospital, or have died.

Case-notes will be most useful for those conditions where it is clear that an incorrect diagnosis was made, or that inappropriate management was instituted. This in turn requires that the information to make a diagnosis and details of the treatment should be available. However notes are seldom structured in a completely logical or chronological sequence, and important pieces of information may not be recorded. Most commonly absent are results of tests and X-ray films; *'for three quarters of the occasions on which X-rays were performed, no report was present in the case-notes'* [12]. Significant negatives, signs whose absence is essential for differential diagnosis, are also often omitted. Even the medical history may be incomplete: *'it is rare to find a good treatment history in hospital records'* [13].

Further, what is recorded may be unreliable: an audit of the management of acute asthma found that in 29% of cases the diagnosis had been wrongly coded, *'for example admission for sigmoidoscopy had been coded as acute asthma'* [11].

Identifying particular types of patients

All of these methods of case-note review require the identification of particular types of patients, such as those with similar conditions (e.g. head trauma) or those suffering adverse events (e.g. nosocomial infection). Identifying patients is not always easy: *'even the death of patients can pass into the recesses of the surgical memory'* [2]. To overcome this problem, Campbell recommended keeping a morbidity book, to be completed by a designated member of staff.

Cases can be identified from one of the many sources which document the investigation and management of patients. Table 6.2 lists some of the alternative sources for identifying particular types of patients. One of the most convenient sources is the computerised record of discharge diagnoses kept by district health authorities, which have been used in the audit of conditions ranging from stroke [14] to acute asthma [15]. The discharge diagnoses may not always be accurate [16], so that any disease group will contain patients who in reality have a different condition, and some patients with the disease of interest will be absent. Although inappropriate cases can easily be weeded out when case-notes are inspected, identifying missing patients is more difficult and will require access to other sources

Table 6.2   *Sources of patient groups*

- Hospital discharge records
- Death certificates
- Laboratory records
    e.g. pathology, microbiology, haematology
- Pharmacy records
- Theatre lists
- Paramedical services
    e.g. physiotherapy, dietetics, occupational therapy
- Prospective recording

of data. One group augmented the discharge list by obtaining copies of the death certificates which mentioned asthma, the disease of interest [17]. McCance and colleagues [18] used an ingenious method to identify diabetics attending an out-patient clinic. They obtained the discharge summaries from the metabolic unit because in their view *'virtually all such patients would have been admitted to hospital for insulin treatment and education at the time of diagnosis'*. Identifying groups of patients can require an imaginative and flexible approach.

ROUTINELY RECORDED DATA

To overcome the problem of missing data in case-notes, and to simplify the process of collecting data, a standard data set can be collected on each patient by inserting a structured record form in the case-notes. This specifies which items are to be collected, and ensures that all the data, such as test results and X-ray findings, are recorded together. A natural development from the structured record is to enter the data into a computer, either by direct input or after collecting the data on paper forms. Computerised records overcome the problem of the unavailability of case-notes and provide a simple means of identifying particular types of patients. Many groups have reported using computerised systems for audit, often in surgery of which the most well known is the Lothian Surgical Audit [19]. These systems are well suited to the audit of topics which are easily monitored such as wound infection [20], waiting times [21] or repeat operations [19]. Where computerised systems exist they provide an alternative source of data to case-notes with the considerable advantages of ease and cheapness of access. Thus they can be used for any of the methods of case-note review described above.

At first sight these approaches might appear to be the solution to the problems of data for audit. In practice many difficulties are encountered. A common finding with computerised systems is a high level of missing data; in an orthopaedic database, diagnosis was absent in almost 40% of cases and information on complications was absent in over 50% [22]. Similar problems exist in general practice: one survey of 1000 doctors collecting data on computer found that only one in three practices reached an acceptable standard of recording [23]. A separate study found that *'in one winter month in 1989, 89 of 548 Minitel practices recorded no respiratory infections'*. Even in those meeting minimum criteria for quality: *'influenza was recorded at a rate one quarter of that obtained from the weekly returns to the Birmingham research unit of the Royal College of General Practitioners'* [23]. The problem may be one of motivation; data will only be collected when those involved perceive a real benefit from doing so [24].

Even systems which have been designed to provide extensive clinical information may fail to support audit. The Oxford Obstetric Data System collected a data set of 250 items per patient at an annual cost of over £82 000, and used it to make some 130 enquiries into obstetric practice. Unfortunately the group were unable to use the data for audit as *'clinical audits of obstetric practice demand more detailed and comprehensive data'* [25]. Undoubtedly the data were valuable for other purposes, but not for audit. Audit focuses on topics which cover particular aspects of care (see Chapter 4), and only data on these should be collected and then only for a limited period of time (see later discussion on sample sizes).

Despite these shortcomings, where computerised systems exist they can provide a simple and efficient method of obtaining at least some of the data needed for audit. But this is not an argument for developing new systems solely for audit. Often the systems have taken many years to develop [26] and even when developed continue to consume resources: one group reported that analyses *'could be obtained by hand from these* [mortality and morbidity records] *within 2 or 3 hours—a much shorter time than that expended on the computer during the year'* [27]. Major problems with computers have also been encountered, as one surgical group reported: the floppy disc drive proved unreliable so that *'on numerous occasions it has not been possible to take copies of data files'*; this was allied to an operating system which on six occasions *'caused the loss of eight megabytes (8 000 000 characters approximately)'*; the software package was equally troublesome *'in the early stages numerous failures occurred, with the loss of data ... a subsequent upgrade, however, resulted in major problems in indexing, so that on occasions up to 25% of the*

1200 records on file were inaccessible' [28]. Most groups will not have so many serious problems, especially if a proven commercial system is used. However the problems of implementing computer systems and training staff to use them should not be underestimated.

ECLECTIC APPROACHES

The methods described above were presented with case-notes as the primary source of data. This is the way they have commonly been used, especially in the United States where they were developed. However there are many other sources of data on health care which can be used to supplement the somewhat poorer quality case-notes found in Britain. For example a study of head injuries in children used necropsy findings and coroners' reports as well as case-notes to clarify the deficiencies in care and to identify the avoidable factors which contributed to death [29]. The choice of source will be a compromise between ease of collection and the completeness and quality of the data from each source. Taking a flexible approach to data collection, by selecting the most convenient source is part of good study design (see Chapter 10).

Sources of data

Sources from which data on health care may be obtained are shown in Table 6.3. Many of the support services, such as pharmacy or physiotherapy, keep their own records, and for certain items these are often more complete and simpler to access than case-notes. For example it might be easier to determine which virological assays were requested and what the findings were by reviewing the records of the microbiology department, rather than examining case-notes. Necropsy reports are also a valuable and underused source of data for audit, particularly because they can shed light on problems of diagnosis and management: *'about one in 10 cases coming to necropsy have pathological lesions that would have materially altered clinical management had they been detected before death'* [30].

Table 6.3   *Sources of data*

Case-notes
- Hospital
- General practice

Other records
- Pathology (including necropsy)
- Microbiology
- Pharmacy
- Blood transfusion services
- Intensive care
- Rehabilitation services
- Death certificates
- Coroners' reports

Official statistics
- Mortality
- Hospital discharge
- Cancer registries

Routinely collected data on deaths, hospital discharge, outpatient attendance and cancer incidence are published at regional level, and can be partitioned into smaller local units. These data show wide geographical differences in the use of medical services and in mortality from conditions amenable to medical intervention [31]. Their main value is to signal topics for further study by other methods. This sequence was followed by an assessment of the use of medical and surgical services [32]. Initial findings of more than three-fold differences between regions in many procedures led to a detailed review of medical records [33]. This confirmed the extent of variation, and found significant levels of inappropriate use, but was unable to uncover explanations either for the regional variation or for the inappropriate use. Further study was required.

In theory official statistics could also be used to monitor the impact of attempted changes in the delivery of health care. However a review of studies which have attempted this concluded that the relationship between mortality and health service provision was weak and inconsistent and that *'in depth studies at the individual level are now more likely to produce information about factors limiting the effectiveness of health services'* [34].

De novo data collection

For certain audit topics data may simply not be recorded. These include studies which involve:

- Long term outcome.
- Interface between professionals.
- Patient satisfaction.
- Clinician opinions.

For example if the recovery of stroke patients were being audited, it is unlikely that hospital case-notes will have the information needed, because patients will have been discharged before they are completely recovered. General practitioner notes are likely to contain comments on the extent of recovery, but the information is unlikely to have been recorded in a systematic and uniform way for all patients. In consequence the required data will have to be collected by special survey, either by a postal questionnaire or by inviting the patients to attend a follow-up clinic. The quality of communication between professional groups is likely to be a fruitful area for audit (see Chapter 4), but information on it, especially when contacts have been informal, is unlikely to have been recorded in case-notes. Instead the information must be sought by questionnaire or direct interview of the professionals involved. Patient satisfaction would also need to be assessed by questionnaire or interview.

Additional data can be collected in a variety of ways. The simplest type involves the completion of a record form for each patient seen. Thus a study of patients referred to out-patient pain clinics used a one page form completed using tick-boxes [35]. Because forms will commonly be completed by clinicians they have to be designed with care (see Chapter 7), to ensure accurate recording and to keep the workload to a minimum. An audit in general practice in the North of England used a double-sided A4 sized structured record in the notes, but found that it was unpopular with doctors and concluded that *'the use of such detailed supplementary records for routine medical audit would not be feasible or acceptable to the majority of doctors'* [36]. The problem is that extended data collection will often be unpopular. A structured record in case-notes is a useful method of collecting data, but works best for selected groups of patients, who are studied for a limited time.

An extension of the structured record involves recruiting patients when first seen and collecting data prospectively at each subsequent visit. An audit of the management of acute upper gastrointestinal haemorrhage recruited patients in this way to ensure that details of endoscopy, management, subsequent rebleeds and eventual outcome were obtained [37]. A similar approach was adopted in an assessment of the management of isolated thyroid swellings where information was required from the out-patient clinic, pathology, and surgery [38].

A source of data which is seldom used, but which can be valuable, is the clinicians themselves. A survey of consultants' views on the management of chronic nerve damage pain showed considerable diversity of opinion on the value of alternative treatments [39]. The study also found widespread lack of knowledge about many of the treatments, indicating that lack of knowledge may sometimes be a major problem.

The essence of these approaches to additional data collection is that they should be designed to suit the particular topic under investigation, providing the easiest and most parsimonious method to meet the study objectives.

Observational methods

A quite different approach to audit involves direct observation of clinical practice. In contrast to other methods which review *'only abstractions of practice'*, direct observation can provide clinicians with *'new insights into their own consulting skills'* [40]. This method will be most useful for assessing communication with patients, for example history taking or psychosocial counselling. Three approaches have been used:

- Consultation video.
- Simulated patients.
- Repeat examination.

General practice trainers in Wessex have reported the successful use of video consultations for training trainers [40].

Although it might be thought threatening, their experience was otherwise, perhaps because it was conducted in a *'supportive, collaborative, and cooperative yet critical atmosphere'*. The video is presented to the audit group by the clinician videoed, and the implications of it discussed. It could be argued that the consultations videoed will not be typical of practice because special efforts will have been made. However this is not a limitation, since the purpose of the exercise is to identify weaknesses of which the individual was unaware.

Instead of recording a consultation, specially trained patients can report what took place. Several studies have found that reliable and valid data on the consultation can be obtained in this way [41–43]. Patients are trained to report symptoms, and to remember the questions asked, the investigations performed and the advice given by the doctors. One study used patients with a stable condition, uncomplicated rheumatic disease [41], another used patients with urinary tract infection, a condition in which physical signs are seldom found [42]. However with imagination the technique can be used for a wide range of conditions: for example *'jaundice can be simulated with make-up'* [43]. This method has great potential for investigating clinical practice, but it may have limited applicability. In one study, only 137 of 442 doctors contacted agreed to participate [43]. Further, because of the special skills and experience needed to train standardized patients this method tends to be one which is imposed on doctors rather than one which an audit group develop for themselves. Imposed audits have a poor record of improving healthcare (see Chapter 8).

For some topics there may be no alternative to repeating the clinical examination. Concern about the under-recognition of locomotor disorders led one group to re-examine patients after their routine medical clerking [44]. They found that although locomotor symptoms were common, occurring in 42% of patients, they were only recorded in the notes of 14%. In contrast almost every instance of cardiovascular and respiratory symptoms was recorded. Repeated clinical examinations undoubtedly offer a powerful method of detecting even the most subtle omissions. Their disadvantage is that the clinicians being audited cannot be told about the proposed study, lest they change their practice. This element of secrecy may make the method unattractive to many.

SELECTING A METHOD

The requirements of a good method are that high quality data should be obtained at reasonable cost. The best method for a particular topic follows from a critical assessment of the data needed. This involves asking three questions: what data do we want? why do we want them? and where can we get them? These can be recast as the three steps for selecting and designing a method:

- Specify the purposes of data.
- Specify required data items.
- Identify appropriate sources of data.

The sources of data were reviewed above, leaving the other two steps to be covered here.

Major purposes of data

The description of the full audit cycle in Chapter 2 revealed how audit data can:

- Confirm that a health care problem exists.
- Refine the nature of the problem.
- Identify the underlying reasons for the health care problem.
- Provide evidence to persuade staff of the need to change.
- Assess the effect of any remedy instituted.

An audit of the management of ankle injuries in an accident and emergency department [45] illustrates several of these uses of data. The topic arose from discussion in which concern was expressed about the management of ligamentous injuries. Patients were identified from the accident and emergency register. A review of case-notes confirmed the problem, only 33 of 220 patients in whom fracture had been excluded had any form of review, and only one was referred to the soft tissue clinic. These findings were sufficient to persuade the staff that changes were needed. A management protocol was prepared, based on the results of the study and a review of the published literature. A subsequent review of a new set of case-notes showed that change had been effected: the number of patients without fracture who were reviewed had doubled; and referrals to the soft tissue clinic increased from one to eleven. While it is possible to find criticisms of this study (no standards were used and no information was given on the underlying causes of the problem), nonetheless it demonstrates the efficient and effective use of data in audit.

Identifying the underlying causes of a health care problem is one of the key roles data can play in improving the delivery of health care [46]. Often the identification will require a different method of data collection from the one which established the extent of the problem. For example in an audit of intravascular catheter sepsis, a prospective survey showed that 45% of catheters became infected [47]. The findings were sufficient to confirm the existence of a problem and to persuade staff of the need for improvement but could not identify the root causes of the problem. This required direct observation of staff during catheter insertion: *'medical and nursing staff were observed to follow an incomplete hand washing technique'*. A teaching programme on correct hand washing procedure was instituted and a further prospective study showed the infection rate to have fallen to 8%.

The reasons for unsatisfactory care can occur at any stage of the diagnosis and management of patients. An investigation of preventable deaths in hospital found that cerebrovascular accident deaths occurred because of errors in diagnosis, most often because of inadequate diagnostic work-up [48]. In contrast, for myocardial infarction, the problems lay with inadequate management. The important question, which is usually not asked, is why did the errors occur? Strategies for identifying the underlying causes are reviewed in Chapter 8.

Other uses of data

Data collection can be used to assist the identification of topics [35, 49]. This can be important when there are no obvious worthwhile topics. But lists of topics are available and many important areas for audit have already been identified (see Chapter 4). It is inadvisable to rush into data collection only for this purpose without considering alternative sources of topics.

Data can also be helpful for setting standards. They are particularly useful when comparison can be made between different units or centres; the target for all would be the level of care achieved by the best. However there are other methods of setting standards (see Chapter 5) which, because they may require less effort, should be explored first.

Almost as important as these reasons for collecting the data are the absence of other purposes which are often, mistakenly, included in audit studies. These include:

- Describing the natural history of disease.
- Identifying causes of disease.
- Assessing the value of treatments.

These other aims are undoubtedly important, but they are not audit, and are not best served using methods of audit. There are a variety of epidemiological methods for describing the natural history and identifying the causes of disease (e.g. cross-sectional studies, case-control and cohort studies) [50, 51]. These methods will seldom be appropriate for audit. Randomised controlled clinical trials (RCTs) are the best, and often the only method of deciding which is the better of two treatments [52]. RCTs are sometimes used in audit but they are invariably difficult, time-consuming and expensive. They will more often be used by research staff than busy health professionals.

Which data to collect

Focusing on the purposes of data collection ensures that the essential items are collected and that the amount of unnecessary data is minimised. Many studies collect some data items because of a feeling that they might be useful, but in the event many of these are never used. Equally other studies discover only at the analysis stage that some vital pieces of information have been omitted. To prevent this, each data item should be assessed against the purpose for which it will be used, and collected only if essential. Once the data set has been identified the purposes are reviewed to ensure that all can be achieved with the proposed data.

To confirm that a health care problem exists, all that is needed is enough data to allow current practice to be compared with the standard. For example in the management of diabetes, where the standard specifies the blood glucose to be attained, only a single measurement need be recorded. One of the benefits of standards with objective criteria is that they simplify data collection. Standards which involve subjective assessment of patient care may require more extensive information on the care received.

Clarifying the exact nature of a health care problem requires more detailed information on patient management. For diabetes this could involve asking which types of patients (e.g. newly diagnosed or long-standing), which doctors (e.g. level of experience), and details of the management (e.g. type of drug, dietary advice). Clinical experience will usually suggest which areas are important, such as: the clinical signs which may be missed or misinterpreted; the procedures which are difficult to perform or sometimes neglected; and the extent of patient compliance with treatments. The intention is to investigate those activities which are likely to be associated with quality of care rather than to document all aspects of management.

Identifying the underlying cause of a problem may require data from a variety of sources. For diabetes the underlying problem could lie in the management programme (e.g. frequency of follow-up appointments or referral to dietician) or in patient behaviour (e.g. attendance at clinic or compliance with treatment). This is a further reason why a flexible approach is preferred to the collection of a fixed data set. Clinical experience and careful consideration will indicate the most likely source of the problem. When staff practices or patient behaviour are being reviewed attention is directed to the reasons for particular types of actions or behaviours. For example, knowing poor control of blood glucose is due to the extent of patient compliance, still doesn't clarify whether this was due to lack of knowledge, difficulty with the injections, or simply forgetfulness. In general, as the topic is refined and the underlying cause established, the types of data collected and the sources from which they are obtained will change.

Estimating sample size

An important question to answer is how large should the audit study be. The idea is that it should be large enough to be able to meet the aims of the study, without being too large so that effort is wasted in collecting data. Curiously almost all published audits have ignored this question, commonly presenting data for a fixed calendar period such as one year. Yet methods to calculate appropriate sample sizes are well known, and are commonly used in other clinical investigations such as clinical trials. Presumably as experience with audit develops, calculation of sample size will increasingly be a factor in the design of audit studies.

The key analysis in audit is the comparison of current practice with the standard which was set: the percentage of patients observed to be adequately managed is compared against the target value (see Chapter 9). Because of the play of chance, even if in reality the target were attained, it is unlikely that the proportion of the sample who were adequately managed would equal the target. Instead the sample proportion will be some value close to the true value, the likely closeness being determined by the size of the sample. One way to look at sample size is to ask how big a sample would be required so that the proportion of patients adequately managed in the sample would be likely to be within, say, ±2% of the true value. Table 6.4 gives these sample sizes for ranges ±1% to ±20%. (In this illustration the term 'likely' means that the sample value would fall within the specified range with a probability of 0.95.) It shows that with small samples the range of likely values is

Table 6.4   *Samples sizes required to yield precise estimates*

		Range of likely* values					
		± 1%	± 2%	± 5%	± 10%	± 15%	± 20%
	50%	9603	2400	384	96	42	24
	60%	9219	2304	368	92	40	23
True	70%	8067	2016	322	80	35	20
value	80%	6146	1536	245	61	37	–
	90%	3457	866	138	–	–	–
	95%	1824	456	–	–	–	–

* In this illustration the term 'likely' means that the sample value would fall within the specified range with a probability of 0.95.

wide. It is only with very large samples, of several thousand patients, that the range of likely values will be small. The range of likely values for a given size can be calculated by using the formula given in Chapter 9 for confidence intervals, but it is often better to ask a statistician for advice.

Sampling methods

Once the size of the sample has been decided, it may be that there are more patients available than required. The question then is how best to select the desired number of patients from all of those listed. Selecting those most easily to hand, so called convenience or grab sampling, is unattractive because the sample obtained is likely to differ systematically from all those on the original list. The very characteristics which make this sample easy to obtain, for example their case-notes happened to be on the consultant's desk, mark them out as being different from the generality of patients. These case-notes might be available because they contained features of particular clinical interest to the consultant, so their management and the frequency with which it was satisfactory would differ from the other patients.

In theory the easiest method of obtaining a sample which does not contain the bias of grab sampling is by simple random sampling. The patients are counted and each is allocated a number between one and the total. Numbers between one and the total are drawn at random, using either bingo-style counters or tables of random numbers. Many textbooks on statistics present tables of random numbers and describe how to use them (some of the more popular ones are reviewed in Chapter 9).

An alternative to simple random sampling, which does not involve the use of tables of random numbers, is systematic sampling. If there are, say, 1200 records and the required sample size is 200, then selecting every sixth record will yield a systematic sample. The only requirement is that the starting point, i.e. in the range one to six, should be randomly chosen. This method of sampling can give a more representative sample if the records are arranged in some sequence, such as date of birth order, because it ensures that patients from across the whole range are included in the sample. Problems can arise with this method, but in practice these will occur so seldom that the method is definitely quick but not too dirty.

Sometimes records are organised in groups depending on, say, year of referral or the consultant responsible for the patient. Then it makes sense to sample separately from each grouping, using either simple random or systematic sampling. This method of sampling within groups is called stratified sampling, each grouping is thought of as a stratum, and has the advantage that patients from each of the groups will be represented in the sample. It may not be possible to sample from each of the groups, but instead a sample of groups is chosen first and samples are then taken from each of these. This is referred to as cluster sampling, because a cluster of the original groups is selected from which to sub-sample.

SUMMARY

The methods of audit:

- Are simply different approaches to data collection.
- Differ in the sources of data used.
- Contribute only to part of the audit cycle.
- Need not involve extensive data collection or computers.

The reasons for collecting data are to:

- Confirm that a health care problem exists.
- Refine the nature of the problem.
- Identify the underlying reasons for the health care problem.
- Provide evidence to persuade staff of the need to change.
- Assess the effect of any remedy instituted.

Selecting a method of audit requires:

- A clear specification of the data items required.
- An assessment of the sources from which reliable data can be most easily obtained.

Good methods of audit:

- Only collect essential data for a defined time.
- Use the source(s) which provides accurate data most easily.
- Use a sufficient size of sample to show an effect without being wasteful.
- Are flexible, changing sources and types of data collected as the audit evolves.

REFERENCES

1. Royal College of Physicians. Medical audit: a first report. London: Royal College of Physicians, 1989.
2. Campbell WB. Surgical morbidity and mortality meetings. Ann R Coll Surg 1988; 70: 363–5.
3. Heath DA. Random review of hospital patient records. Br Med J 1990; 300: 651–2.
4. Department of Health. The quality of medical care. London: HMSO, 1990.
5. Hopkins A. Approaches to medical audit. J Epidemiol Community Health 1991; 45: 1–3.
6. Gabbay J, McNicol MC, Spilby J, Davies SC, Layton AJ. What did medical audit achieve? Lessons from preliminary evaluation of a year's medical audit. Br Med J 1990; 301: 526–9.
7. Rutstein DD, Berenberg W, Chalmers TC, Child CG, Fishman AP, Perrin EB. Measuring the quality of medical care: a clinical method. N Engl J Med 1976; 294: 582–8.
8. Bennett J, Walshe K. Occurrence screening as a method of audit. Br Med J 1990; 300: 1248–51.
9. Shaw CD. Criterion based audit. Br Med J 1990; 300: 649–51.
10. Gulliford MC, Petruckevitch A, Burney PGJ. Hospital case notes and medical audit: evaluation of non-response. Br Med J 1991; 302: 1128–9.
11. Pounder RE. Audit in practice: some reports from those who have tried it. J R Coll Physicians London 1991; 25: 339–40.
12. Swansea Physicians' Audit Group. Audit of the quality of medical records in a district general medicine unit. J R Coll Physicians London 1983; 17: 208–12.
13. Herxheimer A. A framework for taking a treatment history. J R Coll Physicians London 1989; 23: 22–3.

14. Williams JG, Kingham MJ, Morgan JM, Davies AB. Retrospective review of hospital records. Br Med J 1990; 300: 991–3.

15. Bell D, Layton AJ, Gabbay J. Use of a guideline based questionnaire to audit hospital care of acute asthma. Br Med J 1991; 302: 1440–3.

16. Whates PD, Birzgalis AR, Irving M. Accuracy of hospital activity analysis operation codes. Br Med J 1982; 284: 1857–8.

17. Eason J, Markowe HLJ. Controlled investigation of deaths from asthma in hospitals in the North East Thames region. Br Med J 1987; 294: 1255–8.

18. McCance DR, Hadden DR, Atkinson AB, Archer DB, Kennedy L. Long-term glycaemic control and diabetic retinopathy. Lancet 1989; ii: 824–7.

19. Gruer R, Gordon DS, Gunn AA, Ruckley CV. Audit of surgical audit. Lancet 1986; i: 23–6.

20. Krukowski ZH, Mathewson NA. Ten-year computerized audit of infection after abdominal surgery. Br J Surg 1988; 75: 857–61.

21. Marber M, MacRae C, Joy M. Delay to invasive investigation and revascularisation for coronary heart disease in South West Thames region: a two tier system? Br Med J 1991; 302: 1189–91.

22. Barrie JL, Marsh DR. Quality of data in the Manchester orthopaedic database. Br Med J 1992; 304: 159–62.

23. Pringle M, Hobbs R. Large computer databases in general practice—of little use unless high quality data are collected. Br Med J 1991; 302: 741–2.

24. Mumford E. Need for relevance in management information systems: what the NHS can learn from industry. Br Med J 1991; 302: 1587–90.

25. Yudkin PL, Redman CWG. Obstetric audit using routinely collected computerised data. Br Med J 1990; 301: 1371–3.

26. Ellis BW, Michie HR, Esufali ST, Pyper RJD, Dudley HAF. Development of a microcomputer-based system for surgical audit and patient administration: a review. J R Soc Med 1987; 80: 157–61.

27. Campbell WB, Souter RG, Collin J, Wood RFM, Kidson IG, Morris PJ. Auditing the vascular surgical audit. Br J Surg 1987; 74: 98–100.

28. Prout WG, Blood PA. The establishment of a microcomputer-based diagnosis and operations index in the department of surgery of a district general hospital. Br J Surg 1985; 72: 48–51.

29. Sharples PM, Storey A, Aynsley-Green A, Eyre JA. Avoidable factors contributing to death of children with head injury. Br Med J 1990; 300: 87–91.

30. Lauder I. Auditing necropsies: Learning from surprises. Br Med J 1991; 303: 1214–15.
31. Charlton JRH, Hartley RM, Silver R, Holland WW. Geographical variation in mortality from conditions amenable to medical intervention in England and Wales. Lancet 1983; i: 691–6.
32. Chassin MR, Brook RH, Park RE, Keesey J, Fink A, Kosecoff J, et al. Variations in the use of medical and surgical services by the medicare population. N Engl J Med 1986; 314: 285–90.
33. Chassin MR, Kosecoff J, Park RE, Winslow CM, Kahn KL, Merrick NJ, et al. Does inappropriate use explain geographical variation in the use of health services? N Engl J Med 1987; 258: 2533–7.
34. Mackenbach JP, Bouvier-Colle MH, Jougle E. "Avoidable" mortality and health services: a review of aggregate data studies. J Epidemiol Public Health 1990; 44: 106–11.
35. Crombie IK, Davies HTO. Audit in outpatients: entering the loop. Br Med J 1991; 302: 1437–9.
36. Centre for Health Services Research. Medical audit tools. Newcastle-upon-Tyne: Ambulatory Care Programme, Centre for Health Services Research, University of Newcastle upon Tyne, 1991.
37. Clements D, Aslan S, Foster D, Stamatakis J, Wilkins WE, Morris JS. Acute upper gastrointestinal haemorrhage in a district general hospital: audit of an agreed management policy. J R Coll Physicians London 1991; 25: 27–30.
38. Cusick EL, MacIntosh CA, Krukowski ZH, Williams VMM, Ewen SWB, Matheson NA. Management of isolated thyroid swellings: a prospective six year study of fine needle aspiration cytology in diagnosis. Br Med J 1990; 301: 318–21.
39. Davies HTO, Crombie IK, Lonsdale M, Macrae WA. Consensus and contention in the treatment of chronic nerve-damage pain. Pain 1991; 47: 191–6.
40. Coles C. Self assessment and medical audit: an educational approach. Br Med J 1989; 299: 807–8.
41. McClure CL, Gall EP, Meredith KE, Gooden MA, Boyer JT. Assessing clinical judgement with standardized patients. J Fam Pract 1985; 20: 457–64.
42. Rethans JJE, Van Boven CPA. Simulated patients in general practice: a different look at the consultation. Br Med J 1987; 294: 809–12.
43. Rethans JJ, Drop R, Sturmans F, Van Der Vleuten C. A method for introducing standardized (simulated) patients into general practice consultations. Br J Gen Pract 1991; 41: 94–6.

44. Doherty M, Abawi J, Pattrick M. Audit of medical inpatient examination: a cry from the joint. J R Coll Physicians London 1990; 24: 115–18.

45. Packer GJ, Goring CC, Gayner AD, Craxford AD. Audit of ankle injuries in an accident and emergency department. Br Med J 1991; 302: 885–7.

46. Crombie IK, Davies HTO. The missing link in the audit cycle. Quality in Health Care 1993 (in press).

47. Puntis JWL, Holden CE, Smallman S, Finkel Y, George RH, Booth IW. Staff training: a key factor in reducing intravascular catheter sepsis. Arch Dis Child 1990; 65: 335–7.

48. Dubois RW, Brook RH. Preventable deaths, who, how often, and why? Ann Intern Med 1988; 109: 582–9.

49. Irvin TT. Abdominal pain: a surgical audit of 1190 emergency admissions. Br J Surg 1989; 76: 1121–5.

50. Lilienfeld AM, Lilienfeld DE. Foundations of Epidemiology. Oxford: Oxford University Press, 1980.

51. Friedman GD. Primer of epidemiology. New York: McGraw-Hill, 1987.

52. Pocock SJ. Clinical trials: a practical approach. Chichester: Wiley, 1983.

7

Collecting and Processing Data

Data are at the heart of audit. Collecting information on current practice is one of the labour intensive stages of audit. Previous chapters reviewed the data items to be collected and the methods for collecting them (see Chapters 4–6), but did not cover the practicalities of collecting accurate information and processing this in a way which simplifies analysis. This chapter reviews these procedures, beginning with an outline of the principles behind the design of forms to record data. This is extended to review the design of questionnaires, the measurement of health status, and the role of computers in audit. Finally the sources of errors in data and their consequences for the interpretation of findings are considered, and approaches to minimising the impact of errors are indicated.

RECORDING DATA

Describing the design of questionnaires or record forms is difficult *'without appearing to state blinding glimpses of the obvious'* [1]. Yet it is not always easy to design a form which provides an accurate record of the required data, and which is simple to process and analyse. Some simple rules guide the design of forms to be used for data abstracted from medical records or obtained by questionnaire:

- Collect essential data only.
- Use closed questions where possible.
- Develop simple coding schemes.
- Pilot the data collection method.

Essential data

There is a natural temptation to collect many data items, particularly those which would be clinically important. Doing so greatly increases the time and cost of data collection and, because of the increased burden, adversely affects data quality. The information required is identified by refining the topic and the standards (Chapters 4 and 5) and specifying the purposes of the data (see Chapter 6). One way to identify the essential data items is to ask *why do I want this?* of each proposed item. Those for which the answer is *because it might be interesting* will often be in the category of unaffordable luxury.

Closed questions

Questions are usually divided into two types: closed, and open. Closed questions are used to distinguish between a limited number of alternatives; for example *are you taking ventolin? yes/no; what is your marital status? choose from: single, cohabiting, married, separated, widowed or divorced.* In contrast, open questions, such as *what drugs are you taking?* are asked when there are a potentially large number of possible responses which could be given.

Closed questions are best when the set of possible answers is small and predictable, and the answers are simple and can be given without qualification. A good closed question will observe the following rules:

- Options for all possible alternatives.
- Options mutually exclusive.
- Provision of an 'Other' category.
- Provision for 'Not known'.

For example if the source of referral of patients attending an out-patient pain clinic were being recorded the question could look like:

Source of referral (please tick one)
GP ☐
General surgeon ☐
Neurosurgeon ☐
Other surgeon ☐
Neurologist ☐
Other physician ☐
Other ☐ please specify ....
Not known ☐

This use of pre-coding, in which the respondent selects one item from a list, for example by ticking a box, greatly simplifies the recording and processing of data. Whoever used the form would need to be given guidance on the definitions of each of the terms, possible synonyms for them and on ways to handle certain terms: for example would a referral from neurosciences be classed as 'neurosurgeon' or 'neurologist'? Missing responses cannot readily be interpreted and may present problems for subsequent data processing, so it is important to ensure there is always an option for all possible responses. For unexpected or uncommon answers the catch-all 'Other' can be provided, with space to write in the response if this is helpful. A separate category for 'Not known' will often be needed. In the example of source of referral, patients falling into the 'Not known' category could have been referred from any of the sources, whereas patients referred from an 'Other' source could not.

A common form of closed question has a set of graded or ranked responses. For example in assessing the severity of chronic pain the question could be:

Describe your pain:
None ☐
Mild ☐
Moderate ☐
Severe ☐
Worst imaginable ☐

The number of options can be increased if finer gradations are required. To prevent respondents from plumping for the middle, an even number of options could be used to force a decision. Another approach is to provide a 10 cm line with terms identifying the two extremes at either end:

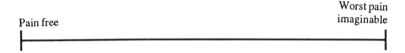

Pain free

Worst pain imaginable

The respondent is asked to mark the position corresponding to the severity of their current symptoms, and the distance from the 'pain free' end is measured. In theory this provides a measure with an infinite number of grades of response, although this may be illusory because of doubts about the reproducibility of the marked positions [2].

Closed questions have limitations. They fix the level of detail at which the information is recorded, preventing the respondent from making distinctions they may think important. This can be minimised by increasing the number of options offered, although the space required limits the scope for this. Closed questions can force the respondent into selecting one option even if none applies, or lose qualifications which might have been given to the response. The possible lack of accuracy of closed questions can be improved by dividing the item into several questions. For example chronic pain is not a single entity, but can affect patients in different ways. Instead of asking one question to summarise the pain, several questions could be asked: is the pain constant or fluctuating? how severe is it when at its worst? how often is it this severe? Each of these questions could offer perhaps four or five graded options. However expanding the number of questions can rapidly increase the amount of data collected and the cost of collecting it. It would be better to decide which aspects of the pain experience were of interest and restrict data collection to these.

Open questions

Open questions are commonly used for items like diagnosis or previous drug therapy, where it may be difficult to list all the possible responses. They are also useful when it is not certain what the range of possible responses might be, for example patients' suggestions for possible improvements to waiting areas. Open questions can allow a more sensitive assessment of opinions and attitudes, because the respondent is free to phrase the answer and convey subtleties of meaning. The limitations of open questions spring from the need to review and sum- marise the responses before they can be analysed. Commonly this involves classifying the range of responses into a limited number of categories. Developing and using these categories is time consuming; processing one open question can take longer than a whole questionnaire of closed ones. In addition, because classifying the responses can involve subjective judgement, bias may be introduced.

Providing enough space for the written answer is an obvious requirement of open questions. But it is surprising how fre- quently forms are printed with postage stamp sized spaces for answers which require several sentences. Presumably such forms have never been piloted.

Open questions can be used in pilot studies to identify the range of possible answers. After perhaps 20 or 30 people have been interviewed, the answers are grouped into categories and a list of options constructed. As a result closed questions, with options for the desired subtleties of meaning, can be constructed. It is best to use closed questions where possible, unless there is a genuine reason for exploring attitudes or opinions. In many instances open questions are simply a sub- stitute for thought and preparation.

Coding

Data are usually coded before being entered into a computer. Coding can simplify data entry and is essential for analysis. The details of the coding scheme will depend largely on the purposes of the data, but some general principles apply:

- Provide unique patient identifier.
- Avoid free text.
- Use numerical codes.
- Adopt a consistent coding scheme.
- Provide a code for missing data.

- Use existing coding systems.
- Prepare a coding manual.

A unique patient identifier is primarily intended to allow the data sheet to be retrieved at a later date. Unusual values are sometimes observed during data analysis, and it is useful to be able to go back to the data sheet to check whether a transcription error has occurred. For this reason and to simplify the handling of records, it is useful to have a separate record for each patient.

Sometimes patient symptoms or medical history are described with a few phrases or sentences. It is always possible to store these as stretches of free text in the computer, *so it's there if required*. In practice such information will seldom be accessed. Often the responses are not coded because it proves difficult to develop a practical coding scheme. Entering the data as free text does nothing to overcome this problem, and simply wastes data entry time. Unless there is a definite, clearly specified reason for free text, it is better not entered.

A simple scheme for coding allocates a different number to each possible response, for example the seven possible sources of referral to a pain clinic (see above) would use the integers 1 to 7. Numerical codes can be handled much more easily by statistical packages; alphabetic codes would have to be recoded to numerical values before analysis. When developing the coding scheme having the code numbers printed on the form, adjacent to each option, can speed data entry.

The answers to many questions have responses of either 'yes' or 'no'. Adopting a scheme such as 'no' coded 1 'yes' coded 2 throughout the form can prevent confusion. This consistency of coding can often be achieved even when there is more than one type of 'yes' answer. For example a question on nocturnal wheeze in asthma might have the responses: none, mild, moderate, severe. The last three responses are all alternative 'yes' answers, and the first is the 'no' response. Consistent coding would be possible if the no response was coded 1, and yes responses were coded 2, 3, or 4.

If a data item has not been reported, then a missing value code is allocated. This ensures that the computer records are the same for each subject, simplifying the analysis. Again it is helpful to allocate the same code, often 9 for single digit codes and 99 for two digit codes, throughout the form. Many computer packages have special facilities for handling missing data, for example allowing them to be excluded from calculations of percentages. This requires that the missing values code follows the convention indicated in the package. Note that missing data is distinct from the catch-all category 'Other', which needs a separate code.

Developing codes for diagnoses, investigations and operations can be a lengthy process. There are many existing coding systems which could be used and some of the common ones are shown in Table 7.1. When choosing a coding scheme, it is important to ensure that it contains the type and level of detail which is required. For example, the International Classification of Diseases (ICD) is used world wide for coding deaths and diseases, but has been criticised because it *'becomes crowded and cannot include all conditions'* [3]. It does not permit coding of severity of disease and is not intended for recording symptoms. Diseases are coded in different ways; for example cancers are classified by anatomical site of the primary tumour, infectious diseases by the infecting organism (i.e. by aetiology), and respiratory diseases by the underlying pathology. For some

Table 7.1   *Examples of coding systems*

Morbidity/mortality
International classification of deaths and diseases (ICD) 9th revision
World Health Organisation, 1977

Read clinical classification
Department of Health, 1992

International classification of impairments, disabilities and handicaps (ICIDH)
World Health Organisation, 1980

Systematised nomenclature of medicine (SNOMED)
College of American Pathologists, 1979

International classification of health problems in primary care
World Health Organisation, 1983

Operations/investigations
International classification of process in primary care
World Health Organisation, 1986

Classification of surgical operations and procedures
Office of Populations Censuses and Surveys, 1987

---

diseases, such as cancer, there could be interest in pathology as well as anatomical site, but only the latter is recorded. To meet this deficiency a system has been developed to code both anatomy and pathology, ICD O (O for oncology). All coding schemes have strengths and weaknesses, and it is best to choose one whose strengths correspond to the purposes of each audit project.

One coding system, the Read clinical classification, may overcome some of the problems of the ICD. It codes *'not only diseases but also history and symptoms; examination findings and signs; diagnostic procedures; preventive, operative, therapeutic, and administrative procedures; drugs and appliances; and occupations and social information'* [4]. It can be customised for detailed coding in some areas and broad codes in others. The coding system is still under development, but it is intended that by 1993 *'the Read codes will be in a position to support all medical implementations within the NHS, including the feeder systems of pathology, radiology, theatre and pharmacy'* [5].

Many audits focus on very specific aspects of care, collecting detailed information within a restricted area on a limited number of patients. Thus any *ad hoc* coding scheme need only cover the items on which data are required, and not include all the clinical features of patients. Whether new codes are developed or parts of existing ones borrowed, the resulting scheme needs to be as focused as the audit topic (see Chapter 4).

It is clear from the above that the coding of even a simple questionnaire can involve considerable effort with many decisions being taken. These could be recorded in a coding manual to be used for reference during the study, ensuring consistent coding. In addition the manual will exist as a permanent record so that some months in the future, when the rationale behind many of the decisions is gone from memory, the document can be consulted.

Piloting

Once the record form has been developed, it needs to be assessed in a pilot study. No matter how well it has been thought out, difficulties will often be encountered when it is used. Pilot studies use cooperative volunteers to complete forms and report on the difficulties they experience. The volunteers should resemble the intended target population as much as possible; for example there is little point in testing a form intended for patients on medical students or house officers, as problems of comprehension would never come to light. The completed forms can be scanned to identify difficulties in interpreting questions, and may even be analysed to detect inconsistencies between answers. Correcting these problems at an early stage can save much effort and heartache later.

TYPES OF RECORD FORM

Record forms can be used in a variety of circumstances in audit:

- Abstraction of data from written sources.
- Self-completion by respondents.
- Recording of statements made at interview.

Each of these circumstances presents special problems.

Data from written sources

The easiest type of questionnaire to design is for abstracting data from medical records. The forms will usually be completed by selected, trained staff who can seek advice when problems are encountered. With case-notes there is a danger that the information may be misunderstood, particularly if non-specialist staff abstract the data. Good training and pilot studies should identify areas of difficulty and may reveal instances of genuine ambiguity for which general rules will have to be developed.

When the items on which data are to be recorded are first specified, they will usually be arranged in the sequence which strikes the form constructor as logical. This will simplify critical assessment of the form, such as checking for overlap between items and for missing items. But the sequence which is logical to the creator of the form will often not be the best for recording data. For example case-notes are often arranged chronologically within specialty, with test results at the end of each specialty section. It might be logical to have all clinical findings together followed by all the test results, but it could be easier to abstract the data if the investigations and findings likely to be made by each specialty were grouped together. The sequence of items on the form should be ordered to follow the sequence in which they are likely to be encountered, minimising the amount of to-ing and fro-ing required. Careful design of the form can reduce the time to complete it and increase the accuracy of the data obtained.

Self-completed questionnaires

Many audits will seek data from patients or health professionals using self-completed questionnaires. The construction of these questionnaires is best approached from the perspective that *'the aim of the questionnaire designer is to communicate with the potential respondents using the medium of the questionnaire'* [6]. The topic of questionnaire design is a broad one, fully covered in several books [6–8] and more briefly in single chapters in others [9, 10]. The concern of the design is to produce a high response rate with accurate answers to the questions. These will be influenced by the way the questionnaire is administered, as well as the structure of the questionnaire itself.

Questionnaires can be sent by post or distributed by hand to patients in clinics or to staff in the wards. However they are distributed, they need to be self-explanatory and easy to complete. A covering letter should explain the reason for the study, emphasising its importance, and describing the benefits to health care which could result. The letter should stress that the responses are strictly confidential and that the contribution of each individual is essential to the success of the project. Headed note paper can give respectability to a study, possibly increasing the response rate. However, potentially sensitive addresses, such as antenatal or genitourinary clinics, might adversely affect response.

Interviews

Interviews can contribute to audit by collecting data from staff or patients on the way health care is delivered. Commonly the interview will be semi-structured, consisting of a series of questions, prepared in advance. The questions need not be asked in a set order, although the intention is to obtain answers to them all by the end. In some instances an interview may be the only way of collecting data: an audit of the satisfaction of relatives with the care of patients during terminal illness [11] had no alternative to interviews. However this method also lends itself to identifying the existence of a health care problem and clarifying its nature. The advantage of interviews over self-completed questionnaires is flexibility. Poorly understood questions can be re-phrased and additional explanation given. This enables more subtle distinctions to be made, and permits gentle probing for sensitive information. Questions which are not relevant to some respondents, e.g. type and amount of tobacco smoked, can be omitted once the initial question, *do you smoke?*, has been asked. However interview based data are not without their own problems. They are much more expensive to collect than data from self-completed questionnaires, as even short interviews will involve explanations of the study aims and a period in which the interviewer and subject get to know each other. The interviewer will need to be trained, again increasing the cost. A second reservation about interview based data collection is the effect on the quality of data obtained. Even with careful training, the interviewer's technique can influence the way the subject responds, or the interviewer may misinterpret the response.

A second type of interview, the non-structured interview, can be of value in identifying the underlying causes of a health care problem, and the possible barriers to remedying it. For example, it has been suggested that inappropriate use of laboratory services could stem from *'routine diagnostic testing, fear of censure by seniors, entertainment of obscure diagnoses by junior medical staff, excessive frequency of repeat tests, and irrelevant test results stimulating further inappropriate testing'* [12]. Clearly, if inappropriate testing is being carried out, the only way to establish which possible explanations apply is to ask the staff involved. Detailed questions would not be prepared, but instead the type of information to be obtained on each of the subjects to be covered would be specified. In part this is because the underlying causes and the barriers are often not known so that questions cannot be constructed in advance. But, more importantly, this type of interview needs to be conducted in a relaxed, informal atmosphere. Since deficiencies in health care are being explored, the interview could be thought threatening, and hence be unproductive, unless sensitively handled.

Questionnaire construction

Obtaining accurate answers is not always easy: the question may not be understood by the respondent; the answer may, intentionally or otherwise, be inaccurate; or the answer may be incorrectly interpreted during data entry or analysis. Attention to certain points can increase the accuracy of responses and improve the response rate:

- Capture the respondent's interest.
- Put questions in a logical order.
- Use clear unambiguous questions.
- Put difficult questions last.

To be completed accurately and fully the questionnaire needs to capture the interest of the respondent. Sometimes dummy questions, whose answers are disregarded, are inserted into questionnaires to increase interest. These questions are designed to increase personal involvement. If directed to a health professional the question might ask for a professional assessment of some aspect of care. Patient satisfaction questionnaires can also use this technique asking, for example, what suggestions the patient may have for ways to improve the service.

The questions need to follow a sequence which appears logical to the respondent, to assist in completion and to preclude the response that *'the fools who designed this don't know what they are doing'*. The structure can be clarified by dividing the questionnaire into numbered sections and labelling the questions within each section with letters, 1a 1b 1c etc. The questionnaire has to fit the expectations of the recipient, including containing all questions which the respondent might expect. For example a survey of patient satisfaction should probably have an early question on how well the patient now feels, even if the auditor's interest lay in assessing difficulties of access to a clinic, waiting time there, or the quality of information given during the consultation.

The phrasing of questions is crucial to the success of a questionnaire. Asking clear unambiguous questions is difficult, and some of the more common problems of the wording of questions are shown in Table 7.2. The solutions to many of these are straightforward if the problem is recognised. Jargon can be avoided; complex questions can be simplified and split into separate questions. Some questions, termed presuming questions, may only apply to a proportion of respondents, and could irritate those for whom they are not appropriate. The use

Table 7.2   *Problems of question phrasing*

Problems	Examples	Solutions
Medical jargon (especially to patients)	*How painful was the gastroscopy?*	Re-phrase to use lay terms, e.g. *How painful was it when your stomach was looked at through a tube?*
Leading questions	*Was the nurse attentive to your comfort?*	Use neutral phrasing, e.g. *How attentive was the nurse to your comfort?*
Composite questions	*Have you suffered from headaches or vomiting?*	Split into separate questions.
Double-negatives	*Do you not think that it might have been better not to refuse the operation?*	Disentangle, e.g. *Do you think you should have refused the operation?*
Presumings questions	*How long have you been married?*	Use filter question first, e.g. *Are you married?*
Prestige questions	*Has the treatment improved your sexual abilities?*	Embed amongst less contentious questions.
Imprecise questions	*Are you satisfied with your care?*	Specify the aspect of care, e.g. information given, waiting time, pain control.
Words open to interpretation	*Do you often have this problem?*	Be specific, e.g. *Do you suffer migraine more than once a week?*

of a previous filter question such as, *do you have a partner?* or *do you have any children?* can prevent the potential embarrassment of asking a lonely person about a family they do not have.

Questions which enquire about social or personal habits which are generally accepted as desirable are called prestige questions. They present more of a problem, as respondents may provide socially acceptable answers rather than accurate ones: '*To judge from responses on questionnaires, nobody watches game shows or soap operas on TV, despite their obvious popularity; everyone watches only educational and cultural programmes. Their only breaks from these activities are to attend concerts, visit museums, and brush their teeth four or five times each day. (One can only wonder why the concert halls are empty and dentists' waiting rooms are full.)*' [8]. One technique is to defuse the issue by starting the question with an explanation. For example the statement *many people find that they don't have time to brush their teeth every morning* could then be followed with the question: *how often does this happen to you?* This might reveal less teeth brushing than the direct question: *how often do you not brush your teeth in the morning?* Clearly this approach, by setting the context in which questions are asked, can influence the nature of the reply. If there were serious interest in questions of this type then it might be best to contact a sociologist or social psychologist for advice.

Questions may create difficulties if they inquire about personal details, for example the impact of prostatectomy on subsequent sexual activity. Questions assessing professional competence may also be threatening. Conventional wisdom is that these types of questions should be put towards the end of the questionnaire, so that even if these are not answered at least the earlier questions will have been. Another technique is to conceal the difficult question in a list of innocuous ones. Bennett and Ritchie [6] give the example which, instead of asking *Have you had any venereal disease in the past year?* asked: *In the past year has a doctor said you had:*

> *Kidney or bladder stones?*
> *Kidney disease such as nephritis?*
> *Kidney or bladder infection?*
> *Venereal disease (such as gonorrhoea, syphilis)?*

The construction of questionnaires is an art, but careful planning and extensive piloting can help to minimise problems.

Established questionnaires

Developing questionnaires is a very labour intensive exercise, with many potential pitfalls. Fortunately there are established questionnaires which cover a wide variety of topics. Even if not completely appropriate to a particular audit, it will often be better to use one of these measures than to develop a new one.

There are many questionnaires which measure various aspects of symptoms of disease. Two of the major chronic conditions, cardiovascular disease and respiratory disease, have been well studied and questionnaires have been developed to assess angina, myocardial infarction and intermittent claudication [13], and dyspnoea [14]. The measurement of pain has received widespread attention and is reviewed by Melzack [15] and Chapman [16]. A variety of questionnaires have been developed, of which the most well known and widely used is the McGill Pain Questionnaire. There are also many questionnaires measuring psychiatric symptoms, and two recent books [17, 18] review the most popular and well tested.

Six questionnaires which assess patient satisfaction were reviewed by Wilkin and colleagues [18], who point out that all were developed in the United States. This may limit their value since *'they inevitably reflect to some degree the organization of the health care system for which they were developed'*. A further three questionnaires developed in Britain are cited by Fitzpatrick [19].

Quality of life measures assess the impact of the disease on the life of the patient, on activities of daily living and general well-being. They do not provide a clinical assessment of disease status but describe the impact of disease on patients. The rationale is that it is more important that a patient with, say, rheumatoid arthritis should be able to feed and dress unaided than have normal erythrocyte sedimentation rate or normal levels of rheumatoid factor. In principle quality of health measures assess departures from the World Health Organisation's definition of health: *'a state of complete physical, social and mental well-being'* [20]. This definition identifies three distinct attributes or dimensions of health: physical, social and mental. Quality of life measures assess one or more of these dimensions.

Two recent books [17, 18] provide excellent critical reviews of the most well known quality of life measures, and a third [21] assesses them from the perspective of specific disease groups such as cancer and rheumatoid arthritis. A WHO publication [22] gives illustrated examples of many of the instruments which have been used to measure levels of health. The measures are administered by questionnaire, and can consist of as few as 5 items or as many as 200. The simplest, such as the Katz Index of Activities of Daily Living, focus only on the patient's ability to perform basic tasks such as bathing, dressing and eating. Some measures primarily assess psychological well-being, some social and behavioural activities, and some life satisfaction and morale [17, 18]. Although many quality of life measures have been well validated, they should be used with caution, as perceptions of quality can vary between individuals. A Lancet editorial quoted Aristotle: *'When it comes to saying in what happiness consists, opinions differ ... and often the same person actually changes his opinion. When he falls ill he says it is his health and when he is hard up he says it is money'* [23].

COMPUTERS FOR AUDIT

Computers can greatly simplify many of the tasks associated with audit. The main uses are word processing (preparing study documents such as protocols, coding manuals and data forms) and storing and manipulating data. Some familiarity with the capabilities of modern personal computers is needed to use computers to best advantage, but a detailed understanding of the technical aspects is unnecessary. There are many good books available which introduce this subject in an entertaining and accessible manner (for example, Anderson [24]). When selecting texts on computing it is essential to choose recent ones—the pace of developments in computing means that what, a few years ago, might have been good advice could now be unhelpful or even wrong.

Choosing a system

The computing needs for different audit projects will vary widely. The starting point to selecting the appropriate system is a clear idea of the study requirements. Some of the questions which should be asked have been reviewed by Frater and Buchan [25] and focus on the information needs of the user. Consultation with those who have direct experience of the hardware and software of interest may also be very helpful. There is no single best solution for all, but some general guidance may be useful. The decision on which computer to obtain will depend on the requirements for:

● Computing power.
● Data storage.
● Ease of use.
● Range of software.

Many advances in computing hardware have occurred during the late 1980s and early 1990s leading to faster microprocessors, greater capacity storage mechanisms, and higher quality input and output devices. The cost of even high performance machines is now modest, and many machines could satisfy the requirements for power and storage. At the time of writing (1993) IBM-compatible personal computers using the Intel 486 chip and running Microsoft Windows software provide computing power on a desk-top which is more than adequate for most audit projects. They will run all the current leading software packages. The development of easy-to-use interfaces such as Windows greatly simplifies the use of computers, and they are now an essential feature of good computer systems.

Commercial packages which can be used to store and manipulate audit data are described in Table 7.3. A number of packages have also been developed specifically for audit, usually based around database software. These packages (reviewed in Tyndall et al. [26]) often include a wide range of administrative functions (e.g. standard letters for GPs, discharge summaries) which have little relevance to audit [27].

The distinction between different sorts of software has become blurred in recent years as more and more features are added to the latest releases. For example, many database packages

Table 7.3   *Computer software for audit*

Spreadsheets
Spreadsheets store data in tables. For example, patient details can be entered as a row of numbers. Different patients are entered on separate rows but each row contains the data items in the same order. Therefore each column contains different values of the same variable, one for each patient. The columns and rows can then be manipulated (for example to generate descriptive statistics) and the data can be displayed in pictorial form. Examples (for PCs): *Lotus 1-2-3, SuperCalc, Excel, Quattro Pro.*

Databases
Databases hold data in a more sophisticated and flexible manner. The analogy is with a card filing system where information that is logically grouped (for example data pertaining to a single patient) is kept together on what is termed a record. A collection of related records is called a file, for example, a file of patients under the care of a particular clinical team. More sophisticated databases (often called relational databases) have facilities to link the data held on different files. Records may be sorted, searched and collated. Simple calculations may be made from the data held within each record and displayed in tables or as graphs. Examples (for PCs): *Paradox, DBase IV, FoxBase, Clipper.*

Statistical software
Data are stored in a tabular format similar to that of a spreadsheet. Descriptive statistics and statistical tests can be calculated for selected columns. The package may include the facility to display the data or the results of analyses graphically. Examples (for PCs): *Nanostat, Minitab, SPSS-PC, EpiInfo, Egret.*

Presentation software
Again usually based around a spreadsheet format with data entered into a table. Used for producing graphs and charts to turn audit findings into persuasive evidence for change. Many other packages also provide some of these functions. Example (for PCs): *Harvard Graphics.*

---

and most spreadsheets offer a substantial number of statistical functions and allow data to be presented graphically. Even so it is unlikely that a single package will provide all the necessary facilities, so that the ease with which data can be transported is one important consideration when choosing software. It is also usually best to select from the current market leaders. Packages from the larger companies are usually comprehensively tested, well supported and undergo continuous development.

Data capture and processing

When record forms contain few items, and only a small number of forms are completed, then the analysis can be achieved by simple counts. But commonly data will need to be entered onto computer for analysis. The data may be entered as completed forms are received, or in batches, for example, one week at a time. Collecting data on paper means that data entry can be contracted out to an established data processing service, for example in a hospital or university department, or a commercial bureau.

If data are to be entered by the local audit group, they can be keyed directly into any of the packages which are described in Table 7.3. A high level of accuracy is essential and this can be achieved in several ways. One approach is to use extensive on-line logic and range checking with prompts to the operator to correct as necessary. Not all packages will have this facility. More effective, and more acceptable to users, is to use a package which allows data to be entered twice. The package compares the two versions for inconsistencies, and requests the user to key the correct version a third time [28]. When outside data processing services are used it is sensible to clarify what steps are being taken to ensure accurate data entry.

An alternative to using paper forms is direct entry of data onto computer by the clinician, during or soon after the patient contact. This method has been used successfully in a number of specialties, notably surgery [29–31]. It is often used as part of multi-purpose clinical information systems which collect routine data on clinical practice. Such an approach obviates the need for paper data forms and separate data processing. However using clinicians to enter data merely hides the data processing costs, reducing the time available for clinical work. Compared to a dedicated data entry service it is inefficient and inaccurate, as many clinicians will lack keyboard skills. Further problems are introduced if data are to be collected at different sites. Either portable computers will have to be used or extra terminals will be needed together with a means of transferring data (e.g. local networks).

Optical scanning provides a method for rapid processing of forms without need of the labour intensive and error prone entering of data *via* a keyboard (e.g. Herman [32]). Specially printed forms are completed by marking pre-coded boxes. These forms are then passed through a device which scans the form contents, recording the data directly into a database. The software can be configured to prompt for additional data or request clarification of suspect or missing values. In this way A4 data forms can be processed at the rate of one per second with almost complete accuracy. Other sophisticated methods of data entry include the use of bar codes and optical reader pens to collect data onto hand-held micros.

The disadvantage of automated data entry systems is their lack of flexibility: all data items must be pre-coded and form design cannot easily be changed. These sophisticated systems are also expensive to buy (but cheaper than data clerks to run) and require expert help. They will usually be beyond the scope of simple audit studies but may be worth consideration if large amounts of data are to be collected over longer periods of time.

Data analysis

The analysis of audit data is an exploratory process which is described in Chapter 9. Modern data-management software such as databases or spreadsheets can perform many of the simple analyses required and can even produce graphs and charts. Yet audit data need to be explored in depth and the findings presented in an attractive manner to persuade people that change is necessary. Specialist statistical packages and presentation software can assist in this process. Regular reviews of statistical software can be found in the journal *The American Statistician*.

Study management

The data requirements of some audit projects are complex, for example data might need to be collected repeatedly on the same patient, perhaps over a long period including after discharge. In such cases computers can be used to manage this data collection process [33]. A database package could be used to keep track of the sequence of visits, generating lists of subjects and personalised letters of invitation. If questionnaires need to be sent at specific intervals, or personal interviews carried out, then a computer system can provide prompts for these activities to ensure that they take place at the appropriate times. However, developing such systems may well take several months and should only be considered if warranted by the size and scope of the study. In many instances a well-run paper system will suffice.

Cautionary note

Computers are not always an asset to an audit study. Although they are invaluable for storing and analysing data they can also soak up endless amounts of time, money and enthusiasm. Nowhere is there greater potential to confuse activity with progress. For all but the simplest of tasks it is prudent to seek expert help in defining and implementing computer systems. Yet this approach too has pitfalls. Computing experts may not understand the subtleties of a clinical environment, and may be tempted to provide sophisticated generic solutions for simple one-off studies. In addition, the claims of commercial companies for their systems are often extravagant: *'enhances the standard of patient care and brings greater job satisfaction to staff'*; *'scheme will become self-financing because of savings generated'* [25]. Yet computer systems are only one element of successful audit. A clear understanding of the study needs and a wary disposition towards the blandishments of technophiles can prevent unnecessary cost and complexity.

The initial expenditure on computer hardware and software is only one component of costs. Setting up the system can be very time-consuming especially if carried out by someone with little experience. Additional effort will be needed to perform vital tasks such as data back-up. Staff training and familiarisation are necessary to ensure efficient use of the system and it is essential to ensure that all involved are well motivated.

ERRORS IN DATA

Data always contain errors. Information may be inaccurately recorded on forms, instruments may be misread, and subjective assessments of clinical conditions may be incorrect. Whatever their source, the question for audit is whether the size of the error is large enough to affect the conclusions drawn from the study. Before this can be answered it is necessary to look at the consequences which measurement error can have for audit studies.

Consequences of error

The main way in which error can affect audit is that the quality of care received may be misclassified as poor when it was good, or *vice versa*. When current practice is compared with the standard which has been set, these misclassification errors could compromise a decision as to whether overall management was satisfactory.

If misclassification errors occur frequently, involving as a rough guide more than a quarter of cases, they will always be important, but the impact of less frequent errors may depend on circumstances. For example consider an audit of the management of bowel cancer, in which the standard was that no more than 10% of wounds should be infected. If defects in dermal coaptation were wrongly interpreted as infection in say 5% of patients, then a surgeon with a true infection rate of 10% might be thought wanting. However if the surgeon had a true infection rate of 25% the misclassification error would be of little importance. The impact of misclassification then depends not only on its magnitude but also on the (unknown) difference between current practice and the standard which has been set.

Occasional errors can also be important when the audit concerns a serious outcome, such as the frequency of avoidable peri-operative death. The target for the acceptable level of such deaths would be low, so that the misclassification of even a few cases could be important. The only safe course then is to minimise errors where practicable, and to be aware when interpreting data of the sources and types of error and the circumstances when these may be important.

Sources of error

Errors can arise from a number of sources:

- The measuring instrument.

● The observer.
● Inherent variation.

The importance of these distinctions is that they point to ways of reducing the frequency and magnitude of errors. One obvious source of error is machine error, and most laboratories have quality control schemes to maintain high levels of reliability.

Errors can also be introduced by the observer. One of the most well known is digit preference in recording blood pressure, in which values ending in a five or a zero are recorded very much more often than those ending in the other digits. This type of error introduces random errors into the measurement since the recorded value would sometimes be higher than the true value and sometimes lower. However even random errors can result in misclassification. If the target for the management of hypertension were a diastolic BP of <90 mmHg, a random error would result in well controlled individuals being labelled poorly controlled and *vice-versa*.

The final source of variation is the individual being measured. Blood pressure is the best known example of a physiological measure which shows considerable variation. However this can be controlled by taking the average of several readings: in an MRC study of mild hypertension, defined as diastolic BP of 90-109 mmHg, blood pressure was identified by taking: *'the mean of four readings taken on two separate occasions and confirmed by the mean of two later readings'* [34].

Validity

One important question to ask of each data item is its validity, whether it actually measures what it is supposed to measure. Validity can be illustrated with an example. Post-operative pain is a significant clinical problem which is not always adequately managed [35]. Ideally one would want to measure the levels of pain experienced by the patient, but there is no objective method of doing so. Instead the patient's subjective reports of pain experience or some proxy measure, such as sleep disturbance due to pain, would have to be used. This may have limited validity because reported pain, or the impact of pain on sleep loss, will be affected by a variety of social and cultural influences. Although these may be of interest, it could be that the level of pain measured depends more on these factors than on the true pain experience.

Lack of validity can also result from inaccurate responses to questions. For example while an obese patient can be asked directly about food consumption, it is likely that the answers may sometimes be a little economical with the truth.

Validity can be important for physical measurements. Instruments may not measure what is intended, or the value may be recorded with systematic error. A classical example is the recording of blood pressure. The Korotkoff sounds will be thought to disappear at a higher pressure by an observer who is slightly deaf than by one with more acute hearing, inflating the recorded diastolic pressure. The consequence of systematic errors is bias, as they lead to misclassification in a particular direction.

There are several types of validity [10] although it is beyond the scope of this text to review them in detail. The general approach however is to ask: *Am I measuring what I think I'm measuring?* and *Is there any evidence to suggest that I am not?*

Reliability

A reliable measurement is one which when repeated on the same subject will give the same value on subsequent occasions: for example the same serum cholesterol result would be expected from a repeated analysis of a single blood sample. The reliability of measurements of factors which can vary over time can be increased by taking the average of several measurements, as with blood pressure in the MRC mild hypertension trial (above).

Poor reliability can be a problem when clinical judgement is required. This is well illustrated by an audit of the appropriateness of caesarean section [36]. Five independent assessors were asked to review 50 operations. In 30% of the cases at least four of the five assessors thought the operation which had been carried out was unnecessary, but *'Perhaps more importantly, when faced with identical information at a different time, the authors were inconsistent* [with themselves] *in 25% of cases'*.

The point about reliability is not that all the measurements should always be accurate: *'There is a danger in studies of reliability of permitting the perfect to become the enemy of the good or committing the error of errorlessness'* [37]. What is worthwhile is estimating the amount of unreliability, by taking repeat measurements, and assessing whether this could affect the interpretation of the findings (see Abramson [10] for further details).

Heisenberg's uncertainty principle

A theorem from particle physics, Heisenberg's uncertainty principle, states that you cannot know both the position and speed of an electron, because measuring the one changes the other. It has a parallel in audit because, if health professionals or patients know that the audit is being carried out, conscious or even subconscious changes in behaviour may result.

In theory the problem could arise whenever an audit is carried out. Staff could modify their behaviour for the period of the audit, then revert to their old ways once it was over. The problem of influencing what is being measured will be most acute if the audit involves videotaping consultations, as cameras are a little hard to ignore. The potential solution, concealed recording, is likely to produce antagonism which could defeat the object of the audit. A similar effect could also occur where data are collected on a structured record in the case-notes. The structured record may act as an *aide memoire* to the clinician, encouraging actions which would otherwise not have been taken. Once the audit is over and the structured record removed, the old habits will prevail. The only solution is to develop an alternative means of data collection, which for the reason given above, would have to meet the approval of those being audited.

In circumstances where behaviour changes can be easily made, for example the quality of recording in case-notes, the Heisenberg effect could be important. It may have occurred in an audit of the management of in-patient asthma care [38]. The recorded level of checking inhaler technique prior to discharge rose to 100% in the month following the start of the audit, but fell again over the succeeding six months.

In other circumstances, where behaviour is deeply ingrained and there are major barriers to change (see Chapter 8), this effect may be of less importance. A finding from many studies, which have tried a variety of strategies for effecting change, is that it can be very difficult to modify behaviour. The only general guidance is that when designing an audit project the possibility of the Heisenberg effect must be taken into account.

The halo effect

Studies of patient satisfaction often suffer from a specific problem, the halo effect; patients typically report extremely high levels of satisfaction with their care. An audit of hysterectomy [39] found that 97% of women thought their operation worthwhile, and 95% would agree to the operation again, if the conditions were the same. More detailed questioning revealed that 59% of women reported symptoms which they thought were caused or made worse by the hysterectomy. The authors concluded: *'our study reveals an interesting contradiction between the number of symptoms experienced following hysterectomy and the high level of satisfaction with the operation'*. General questions may elicit satisfaction, but those which identify specific aspects of care are more likely to identify dissatisfaction. It may be possible to encourage more honest reporting by first agreeing with the patient that care is often sub-optimal when introducing the question; for example *some patients find that they were not given enough information about their treatment, what about you?* or *patients are not told enough about their treatment, do you feel this happened to you?* Assessing patient satisfaction, as with all studies of attitudes and opinions, is difficult and it may be advisable to seek advice from research workers with expertise in this field.

The hello-goodbye effect

An extension of the halo effect is the hello-goodbye effect. It has been suggested that some patients may, at first consultation, report more severe symptoms or a poorer quality of life than is the case, so that the illness is taken seriously [8]. In combination with a halo effect at the end of treatment a large improvement in quality of life could be observed even if none had taken place.

Even if there were no halo effect, overstatement at the first consultation could produce an apparent, but spurious, benefit of treatment.

SUMMARY

Collecting data for audit is often labour intensive, and unless carefully planned can waste time and produce flawed information. Attention to some simple rules can minimise these problems.

- Planning the data collection:
  Collect only essential data—each proposed data item should be assessed and included only if it can be justified; each purpose of the data should be assessed to ensure that it can be fulfilled by the proposed data set.
  Pilot all steps—all aspects of data collection and processing need to be tested to ensure that they collect accurate data reliably and at an acceptable cost.
- Designing the questionnaire:
  Ensure attractive layout—an attractively laid out questionnaire, together with a covering letter which emphasises the importance of the respondent's part in the study, can increase the quality and quantity of responses.
  Use clear unambiguous questions—for self-completed questionnaires and interviews, the questions should be phrased to ensure that they can be fully understood by all respondents, and will elicit accurate answers.
  Use logical structure—the structure of the data recording form should be organised to simplify the collection of the data. If for self-completion the question sequence should fit the respondents expectations; if for abstracting data from notes it should follow the sequence of the notes.
  Use closed questions wherever possible—closed questions, with a limited number of specified answers, are preferable to open questions which invite all possible responses. Open questions should only be used when there is a genuine reason for exploring attitudes or opinions.
  Use existing questionnaires—many questionnaires exist which measure the symptoms and severity of a variety of diseases,

patient satisfaction and quality of life. Using them can be easier than developing and testing new instruments.

- Coding data for analysis:

  Use numerical codes—computer analysis of data can be achieved much more easily with numerical rather than alphabetical codes.

  Use codes which are exhaustive and mutually exclusive.

  Make provision for missing values—there will often be missing values. Providing specific codes for these can make analysis easier.

  Avoid free text—free text can be entered into a computer, but it is seldom analysed.

- Choosing the computer system:

  Be simple—computers can simplify the processing and analysis of data but they may also consume much time and effort.

  Use existing software packages—there are software packages which, when used together, cover all the needs of audit. The commercial audit packages have limited analytical features; statistical and graphical packages will be needed.

- Dealing with errors:

  Identify the sources and magnitude of errors.

  Minimise the error rate where practicable.

  Interpret findings in the light of possible errors.

REFERENCES

1. Cartwright A. Health surveys in practice and in potential. London: King's Fund Publishing Office, 1983.
2. Huskisson EC. Visual Analogue Scales. In: Melzack R, ed. Pain Measurement and Assessment. New York: Raven Press, 1983: 33–7.
3. Earlam R. Korner, nomenclature and SNOMED. Br Med J 1988; 296: 903–5.
4. Chisholm J. The Read clinical classification. Br Med J 1990; 300: 1092.
5. Information Management Group. NHS Centre for Coding and Classification: General Information. Leicester: NHS Management Executive, 1992.
6. Bennett AE, Ritchie K. Questionnaires in medicine. London: Nuffield Provincial Hospitals Trust, 1975.

7. Oppenheim AN. Questionnaire design, interviewing and attitude measurement. London: Pinter, 1992.

8. Streiner DL, Norman GR. Health measurement scales: a practical guide to their development and use. Oxford: Oxford University Press, 1991.

9. Hulley SB, Cummings SR. Designing Clinical Research. Baltimore: Williams and Wilkins, 1988.

10. Abramson JH. Survey Methods in Community Medicine. London: Churchill-Livingston, 1990.

11. Blyth AC. Audit of terminal care in general practice. Br Med J 1990; 300: 983–6.

12. Bareford D, Hayling A. Inappropriate use of laboratory services: long-term combined approach to modify request patterns. Br Med J 1990; 301: 1305–7.

13. Rose G, McCartney P, Reid DD. Self-administration of a questionnaire on chest pain and intermittent claudication. Br J Prev Soc Med 1977; 31: 42–8.

14. Florey CdV, Leeder SR. Methods of cohort studies of chronic airflow limitation. Copenhagen: World Health Organization, 1982.

15. Melzack R. Pain Measurement and Assessment. New York: Raven Press, 1983.

16. Chapman CR, Casey KL, Dubner R, Foley KM, Gracely RH, Reading AE. Pain measurement: an overview. Pain 1985; 22: 1–31.

17. Bowling A. Measuring health: a review of quality of life measurements scales. Milton Keynes: Open University Press, 1991.

18. Wilkin D, Hallam L, Dogget AM. Measures of need and outcome for primary health care. Oxford: Oxford University Press, 1992.

19. Fitzpatrick R. Surveys of patient satisfaction: II—Designing a questionnaire and conducting a survey. Br Med J 1991; 302: 1129–32.

20. WHO. The first ten years. Geneva: World Health Organization, 1958.

21. Smith GT. Measuring health: a practical approach. Chichester: Wiley, 1988.

22. Holland WW, Ipsen J, Kostrzewski J. Measurement of levels of health. Copenhagen: World Health Organisation, 1979.

23. Editorial. Quality of life. Lancet 1991; 338: 350–1.

24. Anderson SK. Computer literacy for health care professionals. New York: Delmar Publishers, 1992.

25. Frater A, Buchan H. Physician heal thy software. Br J Hosp Med 1991; 45: 47–8.

26. Tyndall R, Kennedy S, Naylor S, Pajack F. Computers in medical audit. London: Royal Society of Medicine, 1990.
27. Crombie IK, Davies HTO. Computers in audit: servants or sirens? Br Med J 1991; 303: 403–4.
28. Crombie IK, Irving JM. An investigation of data entry methods with a personal computer. Comput Biomed Res 1986; 19: 543–50.
29. Gruer R, Gordon DS, Gunn AA, Ruckley CV. Audit of surgical audit. Lancet 1986; i: 23–6.
30. Prout WG, Blood PA. The establishment of a microcomputer-based diagnosis and operations index in the department of surgery of a district general hospital. Br J Surg 1985; 72: 48–51.
31. Ellis BW, Michie HR, Esufali ST, Pyper RJD, Dudley HAF. Development of a microcomputer-based system for surgical audit and patient administration: a review. J R Soc Med 1987; 80: 157–61.
32. Herman G. New program for anaesthetic audit. Hospital Update Plus 1992; (June 1992): 96–7.
33. Irving JM, Crombie IK. The application of microcomputer database management packages in medical research. J Microcomput Appl 1987; 10: 211–18.
34. MRC Working Party. MRC trial of treatment of mild hypertension: principal results. Br Med J 1985; 291: 97–104.
35. Kuhn S, Cooke K, Collins M, Jones JM, Mucklow JC. Perceptions of pain relief after surgery. Br Med J 1990; 300: 1687–90.
36. Barrett JFR, Jarvis GJ, MacDonald HN, Buchan PC, Tyrrell SN, Lilford RJ. Inconsistencies in clinical decisions in obstetrics. Lancet 1990; 336: 549–51.
37. Elison J. In: Levine S, Reeder LG, eds. Handbook of medical sociology. New Jersey: Prentice Hall, 1972: 493.
38. Lim KL, Harrison BDW. A criterion based audit of inpatient asthma care. J R Coll Gen Pract 1992; 26: 71–5.
39. Schofield MJ, Bennet A, Redman S, Walters WAW, Sanson-Fisher RW. Self-reported long-term outcomes of hysterectomy. Br J Obstet Gynaecol 1991; 98: 1129–36.

8

Effecting Change

Improving the quality of health care is the primary objective of audit, but unfortunately it is seldom achieved. In part this is because effecting change is not an explicit aim of many audit studies, which instead simply document inadequacies of care. All too often the outcome of audit is general recommendations which are not implemented. This chapter reviews the design of audit studies focusing on the intention to effect change.

Lack of success in improving health care also reflects the real difficulties of implementing change. The delivery of health care involves uncertainties: clinical judgement may be required from staff undergoing training; different specialties and professional groups may be involved, creating opportunities for communication problems. There are a variety of strategies for remedying inadequate care because it can occur for many reasons. Thus this chapter begins by reviewing these strategies.

MECHANISMS OF CHANGE

The mechanisms which have been used to try to modify the delivery of health care include:

- National guidelines.
- Local guidelines.

- Passive feedback.
- Active feedback.
- Organisational changes.
- Disciplinary proceedings.
- Post-graduate education.
- Combined approaches.

National guidelines

Guidelines specifying good management for particular conditions are being issued with increasing frequency. The first formally organised approach to guidelines was the NIH Consensus Development Program, initiated in the United States in 1977 [1]. Guidelines are now regularly issued by the Royal Colleges [2–5], and there is a booklet of guidelines issued by the Royal College of Radiologists [6]. Guidelines can fill several different functions:

- Convey new information.
- Resolve areas of uncertainty.
- Act as *aide memoire.*

The most obvious uses of guidelines are to convey new information to keep physicians up to date in the face of the *'explosive growth in medical knowledge'* [1]. They can also be used to state new management policies in detail, and resolve areas of uncertainty. Authoritative statements have an important role in setting the clinical, as opposed to audit, standards of care. If followed the guidelines can *'assist in protecting the legal liability of clinicians'* [7]. The legal argument is that *'negligence is a failure to do what a reasonable man would have done in the circumstances'* [8], and what could be more reasonable than following the advice of an expert specialist group?

The limitation of guidelines is that, by themselves, they do not necessarily lead to improved health care. By 1986 the NIH Consensus Development Program had convened over 60 consensus conferences dealing with subjects covering *'drugs, devices, techniques, and procedures used for diagnosis, treatment, prevention and public health purposes'.* An assessment of their impact concluded *'the conferences mostly failed to stimulate change, despite moderate success in reaching the appropriate target audi-*

ence' [1]. The problem is illustrated by the Canadian experience, following the issue of guidelines on caesarean section by the Panel of the National Consensus Conference on Aspects of Cesarean Birth. The guidelines were issued *'in response to concern about increases and variations in the rate of Cesarean section and evidence that existing practice was not congruent with available research evidence'* [9]. A survey of obstetricians showed that over 87% were aware of the guidelines and over 82% agreed with them, and many reported falling rates of section. However a survey of the section rates found little change in the frequency of the operation. The authors concluded *'unless there are other incentives or the removal of disincentives, guidelines may be unlikely to effect rapid change in actual practice.'*

Local guidelines

Guidelines may be more successful if they are developed and implemented locally. Guidelines aimed at decreasing the use of routine diagnostic tests and increasing the discharge of patients were constructed in discussion with consultants in four out-patient clinics [10]. Compared with four control clinics the use of diagnostic tests was 50% lower and the discharge rate 40% higher.

Local guidelines can often be developed from national ones. In an attempt to reduce the amount of unnecessary hospital stay, one group developed their own guidelines from those issued by the American Medical Association, specifying the grounds on which stay should be continued [11]. When implemented the *'proportion of unjustified hospital stay fell by 52.6% and the average length of stay on the experimental ward declined from 6.3 days to 4.6 days.'* The benefits of local guidelines may derive from the educational process of preparing them, from a sense of ownership derived from the effort of developing them, and the desire to ensure that hard work is not wasted.

Passive feedback

Passive feedback, sending information to clinicians on their current practice, is one of the simplest strategies for effecting change. In some instances this has been successful: a fall in tonsillectomy rates following dissemination of information on regional variations within Vermont led to the conclusion that passive feedback *'may be a valuable tool for the peer review process'* [12]. However, in general, passive feedback on its own is ineffective. A review of seven studies concluded: *'thus, with few exceptions, passive feedback has been shown in several studies to have almost no effect on clinical practice'* [13].

One of the largest schemes of passive feedback, the Scottish Consultant Review of In-Patient Statistics (SCRIPS) [14], illustrates some of the problems which can arise with the passive feedback of data. The scheme provided each consultant with *'a brief résumé of his in-patient care, some national comparative data and a diagnostic index of his cases'*. The system was set up following the recommendations of a working party (the Brotherston report), not at the request of the clinicians. Although it was stressed that the data were sent in confidence, the first concern expressed on receipt of the feedback was whether this would affect the chances of receiving a distinction award. Several specific criticisms were encountered. As would be expected from the scale of work involved in a national system there were some errors in the data. But although an investigation found that these were infrequent, when they occurred some consultants were sufficiently annoyed to reject all the findings, not just the mistaken ones: *'if an elderly gent is discharged with a diagnosis of twins, the whole edifice collapses with a national belly laugh'* (JD Donnelly, personal communication). The feedback was also quite slow, arriving *'on average fifteen months out of date'* [14], so that the cases concerned would often be no more than a distant memory. The output for every case was in a standard format, and data which might be relevant to particular cases, such as the investigations carried out or the occurrence of post-operative infection, were not presented. The form of the printout was complex and difficult to understand: *'there is thus no doubt that the non-statistical clinician is faced with some obstacles to be overcome before he can begin to use the data'* [14]. Perhaps the most important criticism was made some years after SCRIPS was withdrawn: *'the system was undoubtedly perceived as an external review of clinical practice and was counter-productive in motivating change'* [13].

The experience of the SCRIPS scheme points to some of the

key issues to be addressed when devising feedback. The data should be:

- Locally requested.
- Clear.
- Relevant.
- Timely.
- Correct.

Active feedback

Active feedback, where clinicians gather to discuss the findings on their own performance, has been found to be more effective than passive feedback [13, 15]. The simplest form of this is case-note review, and its effects can be dramatic. One study found a 47% reduction in the number of diagnostic tests ordered by junior doctors [16]. Active discussion of the findings from *ad hoc* studies can also be effective. The findings from a review of the use of domiciliary consultant service in the Northern region were disseminated through regional specialty committees for review by the consultants and their peers [17]. The use of the service in the region over the ensuing four years was observed to fall by 53%, twice as fast as the national average.

The advantages of active feedback are not just that it provides the opportunity and encouragement to clinicians to reflect on and discuss their current practice. Benefits also come from involving the clinicians in the audit at an early stage when the nature of and arrangements for the feedback is planned. The clinicians give their consent to the study, creating a sense of ownership of the data and making them more receptive to the feedback when it arrives.

Organisational changes

The introduction of new systems for patient management can be an effective way of improving health care in the longer term. A simple example of this was the establishment of a 'fast track' admission system for patients with acute myocardial infarction

[18]. The system was initiated because a previous study had identified delays in administering thrombolytic drugs. Patients were being assessed in turn by accident and emergency staff, the duty registrar, and finally the cardiac care team. However thrombolytic therapy was administered only after the patient had been assessed by the cardiac care team. The fast track system was designed to bypass the routine assessment by the duty registrar and to speed the diagnosis of patients with acute myocardial infarction. In the first six months of its operation the median delay to the administration of thrombolytic drugs fell from 93 to 49 minutes.

A second example illustrates the effect of a more flexible method of assigning patient appointments on waiting times in general medical out-patients. A system of *'regularly spaced appointments at 10 minute intervals'* was replaced by one in which *'the doctor arranged appointments according to his perception of individual patients' requirements'* [19], rather as dentists do. Patient waiting times were reduced on average from 39.6 minutes to 9.5 minutes.

One of the major successes of organisational changes is the development of systems for calling women to attend for cervical screening. The value of cervical screening was widely accepted, but screening was done on an opportunistic basis. Population based programmes, in which all eligible women in the target age range are invited to attend, have achieved substantial increases in coverage. Often these systems are computerised and organised at the health authority level [20]. However simple manual systems run by individuals or small groups can be equally effective. One group of general practitioners almost doubled their coverage, from 45.8% to 82.5%, using a manual system [21]. Once the success of the system had been demonstrated, the GPs then developed a computerised version.

Sophisticated computerised systems have been used successfully to effect change. One, consisting of protocols for the investigation of 79 common acute medical problems, was used to try to reduce the frequency of unnecessary investigations [22]. Before the system was introduced an average of 0.65 unnecessary tests were recorded per patient, but this fell to 0.19 after the introduction of the system, amounting to a saving of £1.34 per patient at 1980 prices.

Disciplinary proceedings

The idea of using audit findings for disciplinary proceedings is introduced here so that it may be summarily dismissed. It may seem self-evident that threatening punishment would destroy cooperation and defeat the purposes of audit. Unfortunately some seem attracted to punishment: a recent text on nursing audit describes a scheme in which, following peer review, the best nurses be given pay increases, the poorer ones a warning, and the lowest 10% be recommended for non-renewal of contract [23]. Although the author admits that such a scheme *'would be difficult to develop within the British health care system'* he continues *'recent political developments have made it less far-fetched an idea than it would have been five years ago.'* The folly of this approach has been apparent for some years: *'if punishment is the result of a deficiency, audit will become a means of internecine warfare and a source of division rather than a source of strength and education'* [24]. One of the fundamental principles of audit is that it is carried out in an atmosphere of trust, with the emphasis on developing ways to perform to even higher standards; criticism and punishment are anathema to this process.

Post-graduate education

Post-graduate education, in the sense of formal teaching programmes, provides an essential method of keeping doctors up to date with new developments in medicine. In isolation, its contribution to audit is less clear: *'new knowledge by itself impinges very little on clinical behaviour'* [25].

The challenge for educational programmes is not just to convey academic information but to motivate behaviour change. Experience from the United States is that programmes which offer *'individualized instruction have been most successful'*, particularly when led by *'a respected physician, senior to the house staff'* [26]. In contrast didactic approaches were found to be much less effective. Opinion leaders may also be more effective than conventional active feedback of audit findings. A randomised controlled trial comparing these two techniques against a non-intervention group was carried out to see which would reduce the frequency of Caesarean section rates [27]. The educational programme, organised and chaired by a local *'educationally influential opinion leader'*, significantly reduced the frequency of the operations compared to the other groups. Educational approaches have been found to be most effective when tailored to local circumstances and combined with other techniques.

Combined approaches

Many of the studies which have been successful in implementing change have combined two or more of the methods outlined above. Almost all of these have reviewed current practice and allied this to education, guidelines or organisational changes. An audit of the use of laboratory tests illustrates how the methods can be combined. Guidelines for the use of the tests were developed by a group of consultants and agreed by consultation between clinical and laboratory staff [28]. The guidelines were distributed to junior staff, after which a weekly review of the use of tests was conducted: *'the value of individual tests was discussed and decisions taken on which tests were unnecessary'*. This review combined assessment of compliance with guidelines with education on test use, and as a result the use of haematological and biochemical tests fell by 64%.

Even difficult topics, such as the frequency of caesarean section rates in the United States, were found to yield to a combined approach. Feedback of data plus the *'stringent implementation of existing departmental guidelines as well as the establishment of some new ones'* led to a fall in the frequency of caesarean section in one hospital from 17.5% to 11.5% of deliveries [29]. The cooperation of all staff was negotiated before the audit began, and compliance with the guidelines was encouraged by regular feedback on performance together with peer review. The support which this intervention gained among clinicians and hospital administration led to its success despite the financial disincentives of the policy: hospital reimbursement for vaginal deliveries was $3000 less than for caesarean section, and the doctors' fees were $200 to $500 lower.

Organisational changes can be woven into a strategy to ʹfect change. Concern about the low rate of prescription of thrombolytic drugs to elderly patients led to the policy that *'nursing staff were instructed to question senior house officers when elderly patients with chest pain were admitted and not prescribed treatment with either streptokinase or recombinant tissue plasminogen activator'* [30]. Together with feedback of treatment data the frequency of treatment of patients with subsequently confirmed myocardial infarction rose from 12% to 46%.

SUCCESSFUL CHANGE AND THE INDIVIDUAL

The review of the methods for effecting change showed that some features were frequently present in the successful studies:

- Local development.
- Negotiation leading to general agreement.
- Feedback provided on quality of care.
- Discussion of findings facilitated.

The common theme of these features is the high level of involvement of individuals in all aspects of the audit. Changes in the delivery of health care are unlikely to be successful unless individuals involved want the changes made: *'experience in industry suggests that even the most rational change can be obstructed if its implementation is either badly planned or inadequately negotiated'* [31]. Staff should feel that the audit belongs to *'us'*, rather than being foisted on us by *'them'*. By reviewing for themselves the quality of current care, the need for change will be evident. Finally the impact of proposed changes will appear much less threatening because the staff were involved in their design. The success of any strategy to implement change depends on the enthusiasm of the staff involved for that change.

Involving individuals in the audit is important, but it is not sufficient to ensure the successful implementation of change. The potential impact on everyone likely to be affected by a proposed change needs to be recognised. Individuals often resist change: *'typical forms of human resistance are parochial self-interest, misunderstanding and lack of trust, different assessments of the situation and the proposed solution, and low tolerance of change'* [32]. The strategy for change takes account of four key features which will increase the likelihood of success. The proposed change should, as far as possible, be:

- Non-threatening.
- Perceived as being beneficial.
- Compatible with current beliefs and practices.
- Implemented incrementally.

Change can be threatening because it involves the use of new techniques or equipment, for which new skills must be learned. For example most adults are intimidated when they first encounter computers (children seem immune to this) and it is only with experience that they are able to use them with equanimity. This intimidation will be more pronounced when the new skill or responsibility is presented as essential for a health professional who wishes to provide an acceptable level of health care. An alternative approach is to begin by emphasising the high quality of care that the individual currently offers. The new skill is then presented as an opportunity for an individual, whose intention is to provide the best possible service, to do an even better job.

Individuals often view proposed changes in terms of *'what will it cost me'* and *'what can I get out of it'*. Changes which lead to additional work or responsibility will often be resisted, and unfortunately many changes do involve extra work for someone. Thus the change needs to be be presented so that each individual feels that overall there is a personal net benefit. Again the main benefit is being able to provide improved patient care, so the reasons why this will happen need to be clearly explained.

The proposed change needs to make sense given current medical knowledge. For example bloodletting was a treatment employed for many diseases, and was based on the doctrine of humours. There were thought to be four humours, or fluids, in the body, and disease resulted from an imbalance between them. Bloodletting was the obvious treatment and those of the heroic school *'held with copious bleeding on all occasions'* [33]. It was only in the 19th Century, when the doctrine of humours was finally overthrown, that the practice fell into abeyance: *'bloodletting followed humoral doctrines and finally departed with them'*. [33]

The final characteristic of successful strategies for change is an incremental implementation: *'individuals generally go through a number of stages in changing their behaviour including awareness of the new idea, interest, appraisal, trial and finally adoption'* [34]. Sudden radical changes will be resisted, but those which are phased in gradually, with an initial trial period after which the strategy is reviewed, are more likely to be accepted. The emphasis instead is, why don't we try this to see if it leads to improved patient care? This stepwise approach also emphasises that the individuals have control over the process of change.

The central role of individuals in audit means that care must be taken to ensure that all relevant staff are involved. This can be much more than those involved in the immediate care of the patient; it can include the support services (e.g. pharmacy, laboratory, rehabilitation, dietetics), reception staff, administrators, general practitioners. For each individual, an assessment should be made of:

- Current involvement.
- Likely impact of the change.

The intention is to be sure that everyone, especially those who could obstruct the change, are involved in the audit and committed to its success.

DEVELOPING A STRATEGY FOR PROMOTING CHANGE

There is much more to the development of a strategy for change than simply opting for one of the mechanisms for change, and imbuing it with the characteristics likely to make it successful. The strategy must be tailored to the particular circumstances, and its development can be divided into several stages:

- Create atmosphere for change.
- Identify causes of health care problem.
- Develop appropriate solution.
- Ensure adequate resources.
- Anticipate knock-on effects.
- Monitor effect of strategy.

Creating an atmosphere for change

The willingness of the members of a clinical team to adopt new treatments at the expense of old favourites depends to a large extent on whether there is a *'climate for excellence'* [35]. This means a shared view that, within the resources of the group, their performance will be as good as a centre of excellence. The critical feature is a genuine consensus, in which all the team members have assessed and approved the vision: *'if all the members of the health care team are involved in determining the character of the practice they are more likely to be committed to those ideals and to implement them'* [32]. In this environment, innovations aimed at improving care are more likely to be adopted.

Part of the process of creating an atmosphere for change is to ensure that the audit is non-threatening. Since audit seeks to improve the delivery of health care, there is an implied threat that the performance of some staff may be found unsatisfactory. Even if this is not the case, some may see changes to the current order as threatening. Audit is more likely to be successful if it is conducted in a non-critical supportive environment, for which the approaches outlined in Chapter 3 can be useful.

When an environment conducive to audit has been established, it has to be agreed that the topic chosen is clinically important. The assessment criteria for a good topic, outlined in Chapter 4, could be used as the basis for discussion. When there is such agreement on the importance of the topic, clear evidence that current practice falls short of desirable standards helps motivate people to change. Successful change is easier to achieve if there is a formal recognition that the problem is serious enough to warrant action. Taking such a decision is akin to making a commitment to change, even though at this stage, the nature of the change may not have been decided. Separating this commitment to change from the nature of the change can be important. Presenting staff with proposals before their support has been enlisted may create problems for the implementation of changes.

Identifying causes of health care problems

The key to selecting the appropriate method for effecting change is to identify the reasons why the deficiency in care occurred.

This is more than just asking what went wrong, it is to ask why it should have gone wrong. This is the distinction between the immediate cause and the underlying cause (see Chapter 2). It can be illustrated by the example of the measles epidemic which occurred in Scotland in 1982. The immediate cause of the epidemic was the low uptake of immunisation, but the underlying reasons for this were more complex [36]. Investigations revealed an unfortunate combination of attitudes and knowledge of parents and health professionals: '*measles was not regarded as a serious illness by 34%* [of parents] *and only 44% considered the vaccine safe .... not all GPs were convinced of the value of measles immunisation and an estimated 54% appeared to leave the initiative to parents*'. A coordinated campaign involving formal education of health care staff and a media campaign to educate parents produced an increase of 13% in vaccine uptake within a year.

Finding the underlying cause is not always easy. An audit of appendectomy in two hospitals showed that in one 27% of the appendices removed were normal, whereas in the other it was only 10% [24]. On investigation the first hospital was found to have a much higher proportion of young children and the surgeons defended their operation record because of the increased risk of perforation and peritonitis in children. However closer examination revealed that the removal of normal appendices was largely restricted to two surgeons and '*many of these cases were first seen in the early evening hours and taken to surgery with minimum indications and little period of observation .... it was now obvious that the surgeons' bedtime and the operations schedule the next day influenced the decision to operate or watch the patient*' [24]. Clearly, issuing guidelines on the management of abdominal pain and the indications for surgery would not tackle the problem. Instead, solutions would need to be found in persuading the surgeons to work unsocial hours, or arranging additional surgical cover either for the early hours of the morning or for the planned list for the following day. Discussion of the findings with the surgeons concerned proved sufficient to bring about the desired change.

Sub-optimal care can arise for a variety of reasons including:

- Lack of skill.
- Lack of knowledge.

- Service organisation.
- Patient behaviour.

Lack of skill sometimes arises because of insufficient experience. This is most easily seen in post-operative morbidity and mortality. Surgeons who carry out operations infrequently tend to have higher complication rates than colleagues who carry them out regularly. One of the major findings from the Lothian surgical audit was that higher post-operative mortality following vascular surgery was associated with surgeons who only rarely carried out the operation [37]. A fall in the overall mortality followed when the operations were conducted only by specialist vascular surgeons. An extensive review of 17 patient groups from over 900 hospitals found that, although other factors were involved, the relationship between the frequency of carrying out a procedure, and expertise at it, was a general one [38].

Surprisingly lack of knowledge is not a common finding of studies which have investigated causes of inadequate care. A review of 55 audits on 37 topics carried out in two hospitals found that '*94% of the deficiencies were in the area of performance, while only 6% occurred in the area of lack of knowledge*' [24].

The way the delivery of health care is organised can be the cause of poor care. This includes factors such as shortage of staff, non-availability of equipment and lack of facilities, but can also result from lack of direct access to services. A survey of referral to orthopaedic out-patients found lengthy delays in provision of chiropody services occurred because GPs did not have direct access to this service [39]. Instead the patient first had to be seen by an orthopaedic surgeon and then referred onwards. This study recommended a number of changes to the organisation of health care, including direct access to chiropody for GPs, telephone access to consultants to discuss clinical problems, and training for GPs in orthopaedic management skills.

The underlying cause need not lie with health care professionals, but could arise from the attitudes and expectations of the patients. A survey of prescribing in general practice found that many items were prescribed, particularly antibiotics, tranquillisers, hypnotics and symptomatic remedies, although the

GP felt discomfort in doing so [40]. Patient expectation was reported to be the most common reason for the decisions, despite concerns about drug toxicity and the appropriateness of treatment.

Non-attendance by patients can also be a reason for poor care. A survey at a paediatric out-patient clinic showed that 61% of non-attenders were subsequently assessed as still needing to attend for treatment [41]. A variety of reasons were given for non-attendance including symptomatic improvement, forgetfulness and domestic difficulties. The underlying problems appeared to be insufficient information to parents about the importance of continuing care, together with the real costs to parents of attending clinics. An overlapping set of explanations was found in a study of non-attenders at a dermatology out-patient clinic [42]. Difficulties of keeping the appointment again figured prominently, but illness was also a common explanation. Both studies concluded that additional means of following up patients, by more effective appointments systems and the use of health service personnel, were required.

One useful approach to identify the underlying cause is to dissect the way care is delivered by asking questions of the type listed in Table 8.1. These help narrow down the possible causes, distinguishing between availability and use of services, clinical knowledge and clinical expertise.

Developing appropriate solutions

The importance of identifying the underlying cause of a health care problem is most apparent when designing an appropriate solution. For example an audit of ankle injuries was conducted because of fears that treatment was sub-optimal [43]. The solution proposed, a management protocol, was successful: *'using a protocol can, at little expense, improve the treatment of ankle injuries and reduce the cost of radiology in an accident and emergency department'*. This type of solution would not have been successful for an audit of heart disease in neonates, also aimed at improving management [44]. Here the problem lay with a delay in instigating management prior to referral to a specialist centre, and arose from difficulties in reaching a clinical

Table 8.1   *Questions to ask to explore underlying causes of health care problems*

Was delay before patient seen or treated—	acceptable?
Were the appropriate investigations—	available?
	carried out?
	ordered timeously?
	acted upon?
For inappropriate investigations, was—	the indication not known?
	the test ordered by convention?
Was the diagnosis—	correctly made?
	timeously made?
Were the appropriate treatments—	given?
	timeously started?
	correctly administered?
Did the management involve—	adequate follow-up?
	appropriate use of other services?
	appropriate forward referral?
Were the staff immediately responsible—	adequately qualified?
	sufficiently experienced?
With other staff involved was there—	good communication?
	timely response?
	adequate response?
Did sub-optimal care occur—	at an unusual time?
	in an unusual location?

diagnosis. In this instance the appropriate solution was a diagnostic algorithm, which *'significantly improves diagnostic accuracy and management'* [44].

There are many possible causes of poor health care and Table 8.2 lists several together with the types of solutions which might be tried for each. The solutions are diverse and it is clear that many could be effective in some circumstances, but would be wholly ineffective in others. No solution will be universally applicable. This may be part of the explanation why the methods of change reviewed above had intermittent success, and why combined approaches, which have an increased chance of hitting the true problem, are more likely to be successful.

The problem facing auditors is not just of effecting change but of maintaining it. As Eisenberg pointed out [26]: *'newly learned behaviour generally requires reinforcement to become installed as a regular part of behaviour'*. It may be easier for organisational changes to exert longer lasting effects, by making the new behaviour part of the normal routine.

Table 8.2   *Fitting the solution to the cause of inadequate care*

Causes	Solutions
Individual	
Unawareness of problem	Feedback
Lack of knowledge	Education, clinical algorithms
Inexperience	Training, specialisation, support
Inappropriate drug use	Formulary, ward pharmacist
Human error	Feedback and discussion, consciousness raising, clinical algorithms
Lack of management plan	Clinical algorithm
Defensive practice	Reassurance, education
Entrenched views	Education, peer group leader
Personal convenience	Feedback, clarify advantages of alternative
Organisational	
Non-availability of services	Negotiation with health authority, service restructuring
Lack of resources	Negotiation with health authority
Failure of services	Reorganisation, extra resources
Communication failure	Agreed communication system
Overlong waiting time	Revised booking system, reorganisation, extra resources
Inadequate supervision	Clinic reorganisation
External	
Patient pressure	Explain risks
Patient non-compliance	Explain benefits

Ensuring adequate resources

When trying to implement change, it is not enough to develop an appropriate solution, there must be sufficient resources for it to be implemented. For example a study of children with sickle cell disease found *'only eight* [of 31] *had had three of the blood tests necessary for good care ... prophylactic treatment with penicillin and folic acid was erratic'* [45]. The underlying cause was the the lack of an effective recall system, but a barrier to successful change was the costs in time and money to implement and run such a system.

Perhaps the most important resource is time. Health professionals are busy, and strategies for change which do not make provision for an increase in workload are unlikely to succeed. The impact of any strategy for change needs to be assessed, to ensure that working practices can be modified to accommodate it.

In many instances the resource implications may need funding from health authorities. To achieve this a cogent argument needs to be presented, to demonstrate the benefits to patient care which will result. The audit data will not only indicate the solution to the health care problem, they may also be used to ensure its implementation.

Anticipating knock-on effects

Changes made in health care delivery may have consequences beyond those originally intended. When a new computer system was introduced into a general practice, the partners took advantage of its new facility for prescribing during the consultation [46]. Unfortunately the dispensary staff were not involved in the purchase of the computer system, received little training for it, and were left to cope with the problems it created. One unintended consequence was that prescriptions which were entered near the bottom of the queue for dispensing remained there, never being dispensed. The dispensing staff: *'took all the flack for a teething problem in a computer system they had not chosen ... the resulting crisis required considerable time before solutions were found'* [46].

The complexity of the organisation of health care gives considerable potential for knock-on effects. Thus when planning a strategy for change the possible knock-on effects, in terms of resources and other staff, should be reviewed. These can be sought by asking: *'what other activities could be affected, and who has interests in these?'*.

Monitoring the impact

The final stage of developing a strategy for change is to plan the way in which its impact will be monitored. If a health care problem was thought sufficiently important to audit, then it is worth knowing whether the remedy has proved successful. Complete success will encourage the group to further studies. Partial success, which is more likely, will raise the question: is the extent of improvement sufficient or should further interventions be planned? Planning to monitor the impact of change is an affirmation by the audit group that audit is worthwhile and that the group is committed to improving the quality of health care.

SUMMARY

There are a variety of mechanisms for effecting change in the delivery of health care. Those which are most frequently successful involve:

- Local development.
- Feedback on current practice.
- Staff consultation at all stages of the audit.

Change is often resisted by individuals, who may find it:

- Threatening.
- Involves additional work.
- Challenges conventional practice.

To overcome the resistance, it should be stressed that the proposed change will:

- Be under local control.
- Lead to improved patient care.
- Be implemented incrementally.

Change is more likely to be successful if introduced in a supportive environment. To achieve this it must be recognised that:

- Staff currently provide high quality care.
- Audit findings are confidential.
- Audit is a tool to help staff do an even better job.

The appropriate solution to a health care problem is developed by reviewing:

- The underlying causes.
- Barriers to implementation.
- Resources required.
- Knock-on effects.

REFERENCES

1. Kosecoff J, Kanouse DE, Rogers WH, McCloskey L, Winslow CM, Brook RH. Effects of the National Institutes of Health Consensus Development Program on physician practice. J Am Med Assoc 1987; 258: 2708–13.
2. Working Group of the British Society for Rheumatology and the Research Unit of the Royal College of Physicians. Guidelines and a proposed audit protocol for the initial management of an acute hot joint. J R Coll Physicians London 1992; 26: 83–5.
3. Working Group of the Research Unit of the Royal College of Physicians. Palliative Care: Guidelines for good practice and audit measures. J R Coll Physicians London 1991; 25: 325–8.
4. Working Group of The Research Unit of The Royal College of Physicians. Guidelines for the management of acute urinary tract infection in childhood. J R Coll Physicians London 1991; 25: 36–42.
5. Workshop of the Research Unit of the Royal College of Physicians, Department of Dermatology, University of Glasgow, British Association of Dermatologists. Guidelines for the management of patients with psoriasis. Br Med J 1991; 303: 829–35.
6. Royal College of Radiologists. Making the best use of a Department of Radiology. London: Royal College of Radiologists, 1989.
7. Fowkes FGR, Davies ER, Evans KT, Green G, Hugh AE, Nolan DJ, et al. Compliance with the Royal College of Radiologists' guidelines on the use of pre-operative chest radiographs. Clin Radiol 1987; 38: 45–8.
8. Kloss D. The duty of care: medical negligence. Br Med J 1984; 289: 66–9.
9. Lomas J, Anderson GM, Domnick-Pierre K, Vayda E, Enkin MW, Hannah WJ. Do practice guidelines guide practice? The effect of a consensus statement on the practice of physicians. N Engl J Med 1989; 321: 1306–11.
10. Hall R, Roberts CJ, Coles GA, Fisher DJ, Fowkes FGR, Jones JH, et al. The impact of guidelines in clinical outpatient practice. J R Coll Physicians London 1988; 22: 244–7.
11. Mozes B, Halkin H, Katz A, Schiff E, Modan B. Reduction of redundant hospital stay through controlled intervention. Lancet 1987; i: 968–9.
12. Wennberg JE, Blowers L, Parker R, Gittelsohn AM. Changes in tonsillectomy rates associated with feedback and review. Paediatrics 1977; 59: 821–6.

13. Mitchell MW, Fowkes FGR. Audit reviewed: does feedback on performance change clinical behaviour? J R Coll Physicians London 1985; 19: 251–4.
14. Heasman MA. Scripts: success or failure. In: McLachlan G, ed. A question of quality: roads to quality assurance in medical care. London: Nuffield Provincial Hospital Trust, 1976: 171–86.
15. Mugford M, Banfield P, O'Hanlon M. Effects of feedback of information on clinical practice: a review. Br Med J 1991; 303: 398–402.
16. Martin AR, Wolf MA, Thibodeau LA, Dzau V, Braunwald E. A trial of two strategies to modify the test-ordering behaviour of medical residents. N Engl J Med 1980; 303: 1330–6.
17. Donaldson LJ, Hill PM. The domiciliary consultation service: time to take stock. Br Med J 1991; 302: 449–51.
18. Pell ACH, Miller HC, Robertson CE, Fox KAA. Effect of "fast track" admission for acute myocardial infarction on delay to thrombolysis. Br Med J 1992; 304: 83–7.
19. Jennings M. Audit of a new appointment system in a hospital outpatient clinic. Br Med J 1991; 302: 148–9.
20. Elkind A, Eardley A, Thompson R, Smith A. How district health authorities organise cervical screening. Br Med J 1990; 301: 915–18.
21. Creighton PA, Evans AM. Audit of practice based cervical smear programme: completion of the cycle. Br Med J 1992; 304: 963–6.
22. Young DW. An aid to reducing unnecessary investigations. Br Med J 1980; 281: 1610–11.
23. Pearson A. Nursing Quality Measurement. Chichester: Wiley, 1987.
24. Ashbaugh DG, McKean RS. Continuing medical education: the philosophy and use of audit. J Am Med Assoc 1976; 236: 1485–8.
25. Fowkes FGR. Containing the use of diagnostic tests. Br Med J 1985; 290: 488–9.
26. Eisenberg JM, Williams SV. Cost containment and changing physicians' practice behaviour: can the fox learn to guard the chicken coop? J Am Med Assoc 1981; 246: 2195–201.
27. Lomas J, Enkin M, Anderson GM, Hannah WJ, Vayda E, Singer J. Opinion leaders vs audit and feedback to implement practice guidelines: delivery after previous cesarean section. J Am Med Assoc 1991; 265: 2202–7.
28. Fowkes FGR, Hall R, Jones JH, Scanlon MF, Elder GH, Hobbs DR, et al. Trial of strategy for reducing the use of laboratory tests. Br Med J 1986; 292: 883–5.

29. Myers SA, Gleicher N. A successful program to lower cesarean section rates. N Engl J Med 1988; 319: 1511–16.

30. Hendra TJ, Marshal AJ. Increased prescription of thrombolytic treatment to elderly patients with suspected acute myocardial infarction associated with audit. Br Med J 1992; 304: 423–5.

31. Spiegal N, Murphy E, Kinmouth A-L, Ross F, Bain J, Coates R. Managing change in general practice: a step by step guide. Br Med J 1992; 304: 231–4.

32. Atkinson C, Hayden J. Strategies for success. Br Med J 1992; 304: 1488–90.

33. McGrew RE, McGrew MP. Encyclopaedia of medical history. London: Macmillan Press, 1985.

34. Horder J, Bosanquet N, Stocking B. Ways of influencing the behaviour of general practitioners. J R Coll Gen Pract 1986; 36: 517–21.

35. Anderson N, Hardy G, West M. Innovative teams at work. Personnel Management 1990; September: 47–53.

36. Carter H, Jones IG. Measles immunisation: results of a local programme to increase vaccine uptake. Br Med J 1985; 290: 1717–19.

37. Gruer R, Gordon DS, Gunn AA, Ruckley CV. Audit of surgical audit. Lancet 1986; i: 23–6.

38. Luft HS, Hunt SS, Maerki SC. The volume-outcome relationship: practice makes perfect or selective referral patterns? Health Serv Res 1987; 22: 157–82.

39. Roland MO, Porter RW, Matthews JG, Redden JF, Simonds GW, Bewley B. Improving care: a study of orthopaedic outpatient referrals. Br Med J 1991; 302: 1124–8.

40. Bradley CP. Uncomfortable prescribing decisions: a critical incident study. Br Med J 1992; 304: 294–6.

41. Andrews R, Morgan JD, Addy DP, McNeish AS. Understanding non-attendance in outpatient paediatric clinics. Arch Dis Child 1989; 65: 192–5.

42. Verbov J. Why patients failed to keep an outpatient appointment—audit in a dermatology department. J R Soc Med 1992; 85: 277–8.

43. Packer GJ, Goring CC, Gayner AD, Craxford AD. Audit of ankle injuries in an accident and emergency department. Br Med J 1991; 302: 885–7.

44. Franklin RCG, Spieghalter DJ, Macartney FJ, Bull K. Evaluation of a diagnostic algorithm for heart disease in neonates. Br Med J 1991; 302: 935–9.

45. Milne RIG. Assessment of care of children with sickle cell disease: implications for neonatal screening programmes. Br Med J 1990; 300: 371–4.

46. Pringle M. Managing change in general practice: introduction. Br Med J 1992; 304: 1357–8.

9

Analysing and Interpreting Data

Interpreting the data produced in studies can be the most exciting part of audit. Statistical methods are simply formal techniques to assist in this interpretation. Fortunately, in well designed audit studies where the analyses have been planned in advance, the statistical methods needed are few and straightforward; they will be needed to help answer three questions:

- Is care unsatisfactory?
- What are the possible reasons for this?
- Was the intervention followed by change?

The statistical methods which will help answer these questions are described briefly below. Technical terms and algebra are avoided as much as possible. More detail about these techniques, and a range of others, are given in the textbooks listed in the Appendix to this chapter.

COMPARING PRACTICE WITH STANDARDS

A key decision in audit is whether the quality of care delivered is as high as the standard which was set. This involves deciding whether the proportion observed to be adequately managed is as high as the target value defined in the standard. This decision is sometimes straightforward; for example care would clearly be inadequate if the target were that 80% of patients should be adequately managed, but in practice only 40 out of 100 were. However if the percentage of adequately managed patients is close to the target, say 75%, it is more difficult to decide whether management was acceptable.

Sampling variation

The difficulty in deciding whether care is sub-standard lies in what is termed sampling variation. Because of this phenomenon, if a second audit were carried out it is almost certain that the percentage of patients adequately managed would differ by at least a few per cent from the first value. Repeated studies will always yield different results, even when there has been no change in the quality of care. Audit studies which include all patients seen over, say, a six month period will also be subject to sampling variation. This arises because there has been a choice of period; the patients seen in this period are being used as a sample from which generalisations will be made about patients seen at other times.

An illustration of sampling

If the sex of one hundred consecutive babies born in a maternity unit were recorded, it is likely that the proportion of boys would be about 50%. It would be surprising if the proportion of boys were as low as 40% or as high as 60%. However if only ten consecutive births were observed then it is perfectly possible that only four (i.e. 40%) of them were boys. Indeed just by the play of chance it is quite likely that as few as two or as many as eight would be boys. If several separate samples of size ten were taken the number of boys would certainly be found to range between two and eight, and possibly even more extreme values would be seen. It is known that over the country as a whole 52% of babies are boys, but only very large samples, of say several thousand babies, will consistently give results close to that value. A sample then can only provide an *estimate* of the true value for the proportion of boys among all the births, with large samples being closer to this true value. Smaller samples yield estimates which range more widely around this true value, a tendency known as sampling variation. The amount of sampling variation depends on the size of the sample, with very small samples being subject to much more variation than large ones.

Confidence intervals

The importance of sampling variation for audit is that, when a study is conducted, it is not known whether the proportion of adequately managed patients observed in the sample is above or below the true value, nor by how much. An indication of the likely range within which the true value might fall is given by the 95% confidence interval. This can be thought of as the interval which has a 95% chance of containing the true value (strictly, the true value will lie in this range 95% of the time when repeated samples are taken). The choice of 95% is quite arbitrary, but it is conventional.

The 95% confidence interval depends on the observed percentage, p, and the size of the sample, n. It is calculated as:

$$95\% \text{ confidence interval} = p \pm 1.96 \sqrt{\frac{p(100-p)}{n}}$$

The multiplier 1.96 produces the 95% range; other multipliers give different ranges. For example for a 99% confidence interval the multiplier 3.3 would be used; for a 90% confidence interval the multiplier would be 1.64 (see Chapter 2 of Gardner and Altman [1]).

As an illustration, consider a study where the target was that 80% of the patients with moderate symptoms of diverticular disease should be taking a high fibre diet. If an audit of 30 patients found that 65% were on this diet, then $p = 65$, $n = 30$ and the 95% confidence interval would be:

$$= 65 \pm 1.96 \sqrt{\frac{65(100-65)}{30}}$$

$$= 65 \pm 17$$

$$= 48 \text{ to } 82$$

Thus, because of sampling variation, the sample value of 65% is compatible with the true value being as low as 48% or as high as 82%. Now since this range includes the target of 80%, it is possible that, among all patients, 80% were on an appropriate diet and that it was simply the play of chance which led to the sample having a value of 65%. Equally it is possible that the true value was as low as 48%. The range of uncertainty is wide, underlying the need for large samples.

The confidence interval can also be used as a way of testing the hypothesis of whether the sample could have been taken from a set of patients in whom the true value was 80%. It was pointed out above that the 95% confidence interval can be thought of as the range which has a 95% chance of containing the true value. Thus the probability of the target falling out-side that range by chance alone would be 5%. This conclusion can be stated in terms of statistical significance: if the target value falls outside the 95% confidence interval the difference between the observed value and the target is significant at the 5% level (i.e. $p<0.05$). Thus calculating the confidence interval is equivalent to assessing statistical significance. In this case a one sample test has been performed (described in more detail in the introductory statistics textbooks listed in the Appendix).

The size of the confidence interval depends crucially on the size of the sample. In the above example if 250 patients were studied instead of 30, the 95% confidence interval would have been 59% to 71%. Clearly this gives a much better idea of where the true value lies, and if these results had been obtained they would indicate that the quality of care is significantly below the standard set ($p<0.05$). Table 9.1 shows the size of the 95%

Table 9.1   *95% Confidence intervals of sample estimates for a given sample size*

		Sample value (%)					
		50	60	70	80	90	95
	30	±18	±18	±16	±14	–	–
	50	±14	±14	±13	±11	±8	–
Sample	75	±11	±11	±10	±9	±7	±5
size	100	±10	±10	±9	±8	±6	±4
	150	±8	±8	±7	±6	±5	±3
	200	±7	±7	±6	±6	±4	±3
	500	±4	±4	±4	±4	±3	±2

confidence intervals which would be obtained with samples ranging in size from 30 to 500. The exact size of the interval depends on the true value of the percentage of adequately managed patients as well as the sample size; the range is greatest when the true value is 50%, but decreases as it moves to 100%. With small sample sizes the range is large; from ±18% with $n=30$, and ±14% with $n=50$. Even with what would be considered quite large samples, say 200 patients, the range is likely to be at least ±5%.

DESCRIBING DATA

Audit data allow an assessment of the quality of care; they can identify where the inadequacies are occurring and may also indicate why (see Chapter 6). Exploring data in these ways frequently involves breaking them up into categories, such as type of patient or level of experience of the doctor. Often the results are laid out in tables, but graphical displays can highlight features which might go undetected in tables. The following sections describe some of the more useful types of graphical display. These are carried out by the commonly available statistics packages, and many are also available on database packages or spreadsheets (see Chapter 7 for explanations of these).

Bar chart

One of the simplest ways of displaying the data is in a bar chart. Figure 9.1 displays data on the proportion of patients referred to out-patient pain clinics from general practice. These data are hypothetical but are based on findings from a survey of ten clinics throughout northern Britain [2]. They show a wide spread in the proportions, from 22% to almost 80%, raising the possibility there could be unmet need for chronic pain services in some communities.

Dot-plot

A valuable way of exploring data within categories is the dot-plot. Figure 9.2 shows data from the pain clinic survey on the

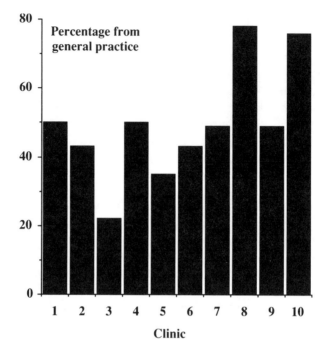

Figure 9.1   *Bar chart of proportion of pain clinic patients referred from general practice*

lengths of time patients waited for their first consultations at four out-patient pain clinics. Clinic A is consistent because most patients are seen within a few weeks of their referral. In contrast the waiting times of patients in clinic B are much more spread out, for which a possible explanation could be inefficiency in the appointments system. The waiting times in clinic C are also tightly grouped but most patients wait much longer than in clinic A. Clinic D shows the most complicated spread of waiting times. The majority of patients have waiting times comparable to those of clinic A, but for a sub-group of patients the waits are considerably longer than other patients. This is obviously a group to investigate further to determine the cause of the delays; for example, were these patients temporarily lost in the administrative system?

Dot-plots allow comparisons to be made between categories. One limitation of them is that comparisons are made by eye so that misinterpretations, particularly when differences are

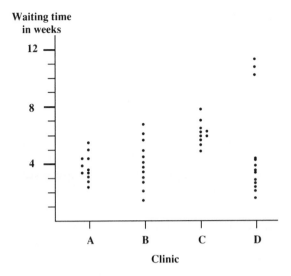

Figure 9.2   *Waiting times of patients referred to out-patient pain clinics*

small, could occur. They are particularly useful, however, when the data have been sub-divided and there are only a few data points in each category.

Summarising data

The data shown in Figure 9.2 introduce one of the most important ways of summarising data, using measures of location. The most well known measure of location is the mean, the arithmetic average. It is clear that the mean stay in clinic C is much longer that that in clinic A. However the mean is not appropriate in all circumstances: in clinic D the mean would be quite large, but the majority of patients have quite a short waiting time.

An alternative measure of location, which tells more about the average patient rather than the average waiting time, is the median. For example if there were five waiting times, of say 4, 11, 9, 3, and 8 weeks, the median is the one with the middle value, i.e. 8 weeks. To find the median the data are arranged in order from smallest to highest. The value in the middle, such that half the values are smaller than it and half greater, is the median. There is only a unique middle value when there is an odd number of observations; for example if there were 21 observations, the median would be the 11th largest. If there are an even number of observations the average of the two central observations is taken; for example if there were 22 observations, the median would be the average of the 11th and 12th largest.

The median value in effect divides the data in two. This idea can be extended to identify three values which divide the data into four equal parts, or quarters. These values are termed the lower quartile, the median and the upper quartile. The lower quartile is the value which divides the data such that one quarter of the observations are below and three quarters above. The upper quartile then is the value where one quarter of the observations are above it. Thus while clinics A and B might have similar medians, their upper and lower quartiles would be quite different.

A second important type of summary statistic are those which describe the spread of the observations, their dispersion. In Figure 9.2 the dispersion of the observations in clinics B and D is clearly much greater than in clinics A and C. One easy way to describe the spread is to locate the upper and lower quartiles, and calculate the difference between them, the interquartile range. The dispersion is summarised in a single number, simplifying the comparison between clinics. The interquartile range is one of the simplest measures of dispersion. The overall range, the difference between the largest and smallest values, is another possible summary statistic, but it suffers from a major defect: it can be distorted by the odd rogue observation (or outlier) in the data. The interquartile range is not affected by outliers.

The standard deviation (s.d.) provides a more sophisticated description of the spread of a distribution, with the advantage that every observation is used. Its calculation involves estimating how far, on average, the data points are from the mean. A limitation of the standard deviation is that it can only be interpreted easily when, as is the case in clinics A and C, the observations are symmetrically distributed around the mean. In clinic D, where there are many more observations below the mean than above, the interpretation of the standard deviation is more difficult.

Box-whisker plot

When there is a large number of observations, dot-plots become tedious to draw and the final product can be messy and cluttered. Instead the information in the plot can be summarised in what is termed a box-whisker plot. This is simply a convenient way of presenting the median, the upper and lower quartiles and the range. Figure 9.3 shows the relationship between a dot-plot and a box-whisker. The upper and lower limits of the box are the upper and lower quartiles and the median is the line within the box. The range is expressed by the vertical lines. The figure shows that the median is not quite in the centre of the range but is higher, reflecting the bunching of the data.

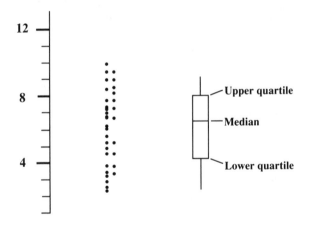

Figure 9.3   *The dot plot and the box-whisker plot*

The box-whisker plot provides a convenient means of describing both location and dispersion. Because the quartiles and the median are marked on the diagram it is quite easy to compare one group with another to determine which has the higher median and which the greater spread. As would be expected, some of the observed differences in the spread of observations in the different groups could be due to the play of chance. There are formal methods for testing whether the observed differences are statistically significant. Coverage of these is beyond the scope of this book, but they are fully described in several of the statistics texts listed in the Appendix.

Histogram

The histogram is one of the most widely used methods of displaying data, and Figure 9.4 shows an example of a histogram of waiting times for pain clinic patients. The waiting times have been aggregated into one week periods and the number of patients within each period plotted as a column. The figure shows the peak at five weeks, and also that there are more patients with waiting times more than four weeks than less. The histogram shows the spread of the data more clearly than box-whisker plots; for example it can easily be seen that a few patients experience very long waiting times although for the majority the waiting times are less than 12 weeks.

The histogram displays much more detail than the box-whisker plot, but it does not show the location of the median or quartiles. A more serious limitation is that, because of their

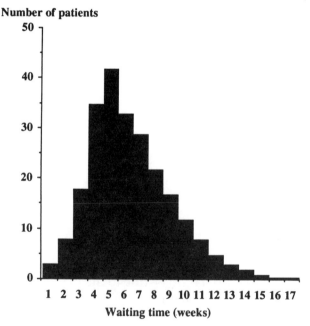

Figure 9.4   *Histogram showing waiting times to first attendance at pain clinics*

size and shape, it is difficult to compare several histograms. The comparison of waiting times at different clinics, which could be achieved readily with dot-plots or box-whisker plots, would be more difficult with histograms.

Scatter plot

The relationship between two variables can be explored using the scatter plot. For example it is clear from Figure 9.2 that waiting times vary widely between out-patient clinics. Among the possible explanations which might be sought for this is that some clinics may have longer consultations and thus see fewer patients, leading to long waiting times. This can be investigated by plotting average consultation time against the average waiting time (Figure 9.5). By convention the variable that we are interested in explaining (waiting time) is plotted on the vertical

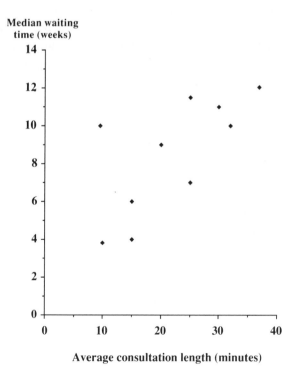

Figure 9.5   *Scatter plot of waiting times against length of consultation*

axis. These data are hypothetical but are based on findings from a survey of out-patient pain clinics. They show that longer waiting times tend to occur when consultation times are longer, suggesting that the reduced number of patients being seen contributes to increased waiting times. However there is more going on than this. One clinic with short average consultation times (about 10 minutes) has among the longest waiting time (about 10 weeks). Other explanations need to be sought, including the possibility of insufficient staff.

DECIDING WHETHER CHANGE HAS OCCURRED

When care has been found to be unsatisfactory, the impact of any subsequent intervention is monitored. The 95% confidence interval could be calculated, and a one sample test carried out, to see if care is still significantly below the standard. But it would also be valuable to know whether there has been a significant improvement in care since the previous survey. For example, suppose that an audit of 250 patients with moderate symptoms of diverticular disease showed that only 65% were on a high fibre diet. This might lead to an intervention in which patients were given an information pack on their disease which emphasised the importance of fibre and contained recipes for attractive meals with a high fibre content. If a second audit of 250 patients showed that 75% of patients were now on an appropriate diet, does this represent a significant increase? or could the increase from the first value have been due simply to chance?

The size of the observed increase in the proportion of patients on an appropriate diet, 10%, will be subject to sampling variation. As there are now two samples involved, each will contribute towards the variability of the observed increase. As with the one sample test, the approach is to estimate the interval which is likely to contain the true value of the increase. The calculation is only slightly more complex. If p_1 is the proportion from the first audit on an appropriate diet (using a sample size n_1), and p_2 is the proportion from the second (with sample size n_2), then the difference between the two proportions is p_2-p_1. Call this p_d. Thus, in this example, $p_d=10\%$ and $n_1=n_2=250$.

The range within which the true difference is likely to lie, the 95% confidence interval for p_d, is given by:

$$p_d \pm 1.96 \sqrt{\frac{p_1(100-p_1)}{n_1} + \frac{p_2(100-p_2)}{n_2}}$$

$$10 \pm 1.96 \sqrt{\frac{65(100-65)}{250} + \frac{75(100-75)}{250}}$$

$$= 10 \pm 8.0$$

This means that the true difference is likely to be somewhere in the range from 2% to 18%. The conclusion is that it is unlikely that the true difference was zero, that there is indeed a statistically significant improvement in the diets of patients with diverticular disease. Because the chance of the true value lying outside the 95% confidence interval can be regarded as <5%, the result of this two sample test is described as being significant at the 5% level.

PITFALLS OF INTERPRETATION

Audit data are observational and in consequence are subject to numerous biases which, if not appreciated, could lead to incorrect interpretation of the findings. For example, if it were found that the patients of one consultant obstetrician had on average much longer in-patient stays than those of colleagues', this would not necessarily mean that inadequate care was being delivered. Alternative explanations, such as case-mix (see below), need to be ruled out before such a conclusion can be drawn. This section reviews some of the pitfalls facing the interpretation of audit findings. The related problem of errors in the data themselves was reviewed in Chapter 7.

Misleading mean

The mean, or arithmetic average, is a useful way of summarising data, but it can be misleading. The classic example of this concerns mean salaries. If it was found that the mean salary of those working in a clinic was, say, £23 000, then this might seem an attractive place to work. What this figure conceals is that the three clerical staff earn about £10 000 a year, and the four nursing staff on average £15 000, and the three junior doctors about £21 000. How can all these staff earn less than the mean salary? The reason is that the two consultants have merit awards and earn over £60 000, pushing up the overall mean. The presence of a few high values distorts the mean. The problem is commonly encountered when time intervals are being studied: a few patients will have had very long waiting times or long inpatient stays so the mean would be high. This type of problem is easily spotted if the data are plotted graphically. The alternative is to use the median, which gives a better indication of the average person. In the example of salaries the median would be £15 000.

Too small a sample

Because of sampling variation, small samples can give misleading results. This is perhaps most evident when percentages are calculated. A sample of 20 which yielded a percentage of 50% would have a 95% confidence interval of 28 to 72. As a general rule percentages should seldom be calculated for samples of less than 50, and should be interpreted with caution for samples of less than 200.

Regression to the mean

Many biological measurements, like blood pressure or serum triglycerides, vary over a wide range during the day. When a single measurement is taken on a group of individuals some will, by chance, have high values. If a second measurement is taken, many of those individuals with initial high values are likely to have lower ones on the second occasion. Often the more extreme the initial value, the larger the apparent 'fall' to the second value. This phenomenon is referred to as regression to the mean, describing the tendency for an individual with an initial extreme value to be closer to the group average when measured again. Because of this the amount of change between two measurements will often appear strongly related to the initial value. A review of the analytical methods which can be used to overcome this problem is given by Hayes [3].

Contemporaneous changes

A good example of the dangers of comparing changes over time is given in a paper by Gibbons and Davis [4]. This showed that the salaries of protestant ministers in Canada rose in concert with the price of beer. Two possible inferences—that ministers obtained pay increases to maintain a high beer consumption, or that the brewers took advantage of the increasing salaries of their main customers (ministers) to raise prices—could be dismissed in favour of inflation being the root cause of both trends.

When an audit shows that improvements in care have occurred following an intervention, this need not necessarily be due to the intervention. An audit of the uptake of cervical smears in general practice found that, following feedback of information on current practice, the proportion of women who had had a smear test in the previous five years rose from 49% to 69% [5]. However the author thought that this was not due to the audit but *probably represents a more general trend within primary care*. However an audit of the uptake of immunisation against measles was less circumspect in its conclusions [6]. The study showed that in a health district with low uptake rates there was a marked increase in uptake following feedback on immunisation rates. But neighbouring districts which received no feedback also showed marked increases. During the first two years of feedback the target district remained one of the lowest in the region. Unfortunately the author did not consider alternative explanations, but concluded that the increase in immunisation rates in the district occurred *probably because data on uptake were collected and reported back to primary health care teams*.

From *a* to *b*

Trends over time are one example of the difficulty of interpreting associations. Showing that *a* is related to *b* does not mean that one causes the other. Even when variables are causally related, it does not follow that changing one will change the other. Height and weight may be causally related but that does not mean that the way to become tall is first to become obese.

Case-mix

The nature of patients seen by a particular doctor or at a particular clinic will be influenced by a variety of factors including: the specialist interests of clinic staff; the availability of services within the clinic; the views of referring physicians; the other services available locally; and the catchment area of the clinic. These factors will almost inevitably influence the mix of patients seen in terms of length and severity of disease. This presents a major difficulty for comparing audit findings between individuals or groups. A comparison of the mortality rates in paediatric intensive care units provides a good example [7]. The overall mortality of three specialist centres was found to be 23.4%, compared to only 6.0% in 71 non-specialist centres, raising the paradoxical possibility that the specialist centres provided poorer care. However the specialist centres received many more severely ill children, and when this was taken into account the pattern was reversed and the specialist centres did better. Factors related to case severity contributed to this reversal; for example at admission, 22% of patients seen in the specialist centres were judged to have a greater that 50% risk of death, whereas only 3% of patients at the non-specialist centres were at this high risk of dying.

Case-mix differences will not only affect comparisons between individuals or centres, they can also influence the apparent performance of individuals over time. It is easy to see how the employment of a new member of staff or the opening of a new specialist centre could change the mix of patients seen. If this type of change occurred it could invalidate conclusions of whether an intervention had improved care compared to its previous level.

In audit the possibility of case-mix effects should always be suspected and, where they exist, steps taken in the analysis to control their effect. The paediatric example suggests one approach, that patients be grouped by disease severity and the analysis be performed separately on each group. In practice case-mix is a much more general phenomenon than disease severity. For example, if the topic were post-operative wound infection, account would have to be taken of factors like length of pre-operative stay, nature of pre-operative preparation, and type and duration of operation, all of which may influence wound infection rate [8]. If the topic were the use of a particular investigation, then patients would be arranged by diagnostic group and within group by presence of other diagnostic signs. The key factors to assess when investigating case-mix will depend on the topic in hand.

THE STRENGTH OF AUDIT

The limitations of audit studies mean that they cannot be used to decide which is the better of two treatments. The excellent book by Pocock [9] reviews the arguments why treatments can only be compared validly in a randomised controlled clinical trial. Yet audits of outcome are often used to assess the quality of care, leading to conclusions like: *'the patients managed in this unit did better than those in that unit'*. Are these conclusions warranted? The answer is far from clear. The observed differences in outcome may be real, but audit studies do not aim to provide definite proof that they occurred because of poor management. What audit does is to identify potential deficiencies in care so that possible underlying causes for them may be investigated. Finding underlying causes adds plausibility to the conclusion; for example poorer management could be due to lack of support services, inexperience, or lack of knowledge. But the existence of such explanations is not sufficient for proof of poor care. The final test is to change the underlying cause and continue monitoring to see if the predicted improvement in management occurs. Such an improvement adds support to the conclusion that there was a deficiency in health care which was capable of remedy. Even then, there are still other possible explanations why initially care was apparently poor and why it has now improved. There could have been changes in other services which changed referral patterns leading to changes in case-mix. Alternatively contemporaneous changes within a unit could have been responsible for the observed improvements.

The strength of audit is that there is a triad of support: observational evidence of a deficiency; a plausible underlying cause; and an improvement achieved by directing efforts at the underlying cause. This still does not provide proof of cause and effect. For audit this is not a problem. If care were initially found to be poor, but subsequently was shown to have improved to a satisfactory level, then the aims of the audit would have been achieved. The question of whether this was a direct or indirect result of the audit or was due to some extraneous cause is only of academic interest. It would be comforting to think the audit was responsible, but good audit does not require formal proof: it only requires that high quality care be delivered.

SUMMARY

The primary statistical analysis in audit is deciding whether the observed quality of care is up to the standard which has been set. This involves a one sample test on proportions. Deciding whether care has improved following an intervention involves a two sample test on proportions. The other statistical methods concern ways of describing or displaying data so they may be more easily understood. Because they are observational, rather than experimental, audit data are subject to numerous biases, and must be interpreted with care.

REFERENCES

1. Gardner MJ, Altman DJ. Statistics with confidence. London: British Medical Journal, 1990.
2. Davies HTO, Crombie IK, Macrae WA, Rogers KM. Pain clinic patients in northern Britain. The Pain Clinic 1992; 5: 129–35.

3. Hayes RJ. Methods for assessing whether change depends on initial value. Stats in Med 1988; 7: 915–27.
4. Gibbons RD, Davis JM. The price of beer and the salaries of protestant ministers: analysis and display of longitudinal psychiatric data. Arch Gen Psychiatry 1984; 41: 1183–4.
5. Wilson A. Cervical cytology in the Vale of Trent faculty of the Royal College of General Practitioners, 1985–8. Br Med J 1990; 300: 376–8.
6. Colver AF. Health surveillance of pre-school children: four years experience. Br Med J 1990; 300: 1246–8.
7. Pollack MM, Alexander SR, Clarke N, Ruttiman UE, Tesselaar HM, Bachulis AC. Improved outcome from tertiary center pediatric intensive care: a statewide comparison of tertiary and nontertiary care facilities. Crit Care Med 1991; 19: 150–9.
8. Cruse PJE, Foord R. The epidemiology of wound infection. Surg Clin North Am 1980; 60: 27–40.
9. Pocock SJ. Clinical trials: a practical approach. Chichester: Wiley, 1983.

APPENDIX: TEXTBOOKS ON STATISTICS

These books have been arranged in categories from elementary to advanced. Short notes on some of the books are given to indicate the style, purpose and level of difficulty.

Elementary

How to lie with statistics, D. Huff. London, Gollanz, 1954.
Humorous introduction to important statistical concepts and common pitfalls.

Facts from figures, M.J. Morony. London, Penguin, 1951.
Clear and interesting introduction to many statistical concepts, to methods of summarising and describing data, and to some statistical tests.

Statistics without tears, D. Rowntree. London, Penguin, 1991.
A good introductory text, well described by its subtitle: a primer for non-mathematicians.

Simple

Statistics at square one, T.D.V. Swinscow. London, BMJ, 1983.
Simple description of how to carry out basic statistical methods using a pocket calculator. Very little algebra is used, and clear explanations are given.

Medical statistics on microcomputers, R.A. Brown, J. Swanson Beck. London, BMJ, 1990.
Clear description of approaches to data description and analysis. As the title implies, the book is designed for use with a statistics package on a microcomputer. This enables it to avoid formulae and to concentrate on the interpretation of findings.

More comprehensive

Slightly more advanced texts which use some algebra. They present methods of describing and summarising data, as well as a range of statistical tests.

An introduction to medical statistics, M. Bland. Oxford, OUP, 1987.
Medical statistics: a common-sense approach, M.J. Campbell, D. Machin. Chichester, Wiley, 1990.

Practical statistics for medical research, D.G. Altman. London, Chapman & Hall, 1991.

Statistics for health management and research, M. Woodward, L.M.A. Francis. London, Arnold, 1988.

Interpretation and uses of medical statistics, L.E. Daly, G.J. Bourke, J. McGilvary. Oxford, Blackwell, 1991.

Confidence intervals

Statistics with confidence, M.J. Gardner, D.G. Altman. London, BMJ, 1990.
A review of methods of obtaining confidence intervals for a variety of summary statistics, e.g. mean, median, proportions and correlation coefficients.

More advanced

Texts which present some more specialised statistical methods. Despite being advanced they are clearly written to be understood by the non-mathematician.

Statistical methods for medical investigations, B.S. Everitt. London, Arnold, 1989.

The analysis of contingency tables, B.S. Everitt. London, Chapman & Hall, 1977.

Non-parametric statistics

Non-parametric statistical tests are those which do not assume that the data follow a normal distribution or some other specified distribution (e.g. Poisson or binomial). These tests are ideally suited for data which are organised in rank order.

Nonparametric statistics, S. Seigel, N.J. Catellan. New York, McGraw-Hill, 1988.

Introduction to statistics: a nonparametric approach for the social sciences, C. Leach. Chichester, Wiley, 1979.

10

Designing Audit Studies

Effective audit needs good study design. Previous chapters have reviewed the principles of audit, providing a guide to each of the steps in the audit cycle. This chapter brings together the salient points of these earlier chapters, to produce a step-by-step guide to the design of audit studies.

The importance of study design is such that it is the subject of several books, of which two recent excellent ones are Abramson [1] and Hulley and Cummings [2]. The design of audit studies presents particular challenges because it seeks to bring together groups of health professionals who will monitor the care they give and improve it should it be found wanting. Audit is much more than simply the collection and analysis of data, and the design of audit studies needs to separate the collection of data from the activities involved in bringing about change. Thus this chapter first reviews the design of audit, and then reviews the design needed for data collection.

PLANNING THE STUDY

The aim of study design is to produce audits which are simple and cheap, and which bring about improvements in health care delivery with the least fuss in the shortest possible time. Phrased in this way it is clear that careful planning is essential. Although data collection can be undertaken with little preparation, this is seldom advisable: *'if he* [the investigator] *concerns himself with a problem without theoretical or practical significance, his findings may serve no end but self-gratification; only in this instance may sound planning be unnecessary'* [1].

Planning a study involves asking certain key questions:

- What do we want to do?
- Why do we want to do it?
- What is already known?
- How do we achieve our aims?

Many audits begin with small groups who have general ideas about areas which could be audited. Designing effective audit requires these general ideas to be translated into specific study details. This is best begun by clarifying the rationale behind the audit; by providing answers to the first three questions. The answer to the fourth question will involve a review of each of the stages of the audit cycle.

The conduct of an audit can be thought of as occurring in five stages, differentiated by the activities being undertaken:

- Set up the audit group.
- Select a topic.
- Set standards.
- Observe current practice.
- Implement change.

Thus the design of the study needs to focus on each of these in turn. A hypothetical example of an audit of the management of stroke patients illustrates this process, showing how a clear assessment of each of these stages during planning leads to a practical project.

A planning example

A consultant geriatrician is unhappy about the management of stroke patients and sets up an audit group with junior doctors and nursing staff. They realise that *management* is too broad an area: it includes topics such as timeliness of diagnosis; use of investigations; referral to rehabilitation; and subsequent morbidity or mortality. A more specific topic is proposed: the appropriate and timely referral of patients to rehabilitation. It is selected because it meets many of the criteria of a good topic: it is a common activity which can make an important contribution to patient outcome and has major implications for the long term cost of patient management. Representatives from physiotherapy, speech therapy and occupational therapy are invited to join the audit group. All agree that the topic is important.

To confirm that the problem is real, a review of the case-notes of stroke patients is suggested. Because of doubts that details of referral may not always be recorded in the case-notes, additional data on referral are to be collected from the records held by the rehabilitation departments. It is recognised that for some patients the case-notes might not contain enough information to decide whether the patient should have been referred. This is not thought to be a problem because this stage of the audit is not trying to estimate precisely the proportion not referred, merely to establish that some patients who should have been referred were not. For the purposes of planning it is assumed that some relevant patients were found not to have been referred.

After discussion it is agreed that the standard set should be that 90% of patients, for whom referral was appropriate, should have been referred. It is thought likely that the initial case-note review will show that the necessary clinical information to decide on appropriateness is not always contained in the case-notes. Thus the proposed method of data collection to compare current practice with the standard needs to be modified: a structured record will be inserted in the case-notes to ensure the relevant data are recorded.

A consideration of how change could be effected suggests that the best strategy will depend on why some patients are not being referred. One likely explanation is that staff sometimes do not recognise the potential for rehabilitation, and hence that guidelines on referral practice might need to be issued. It is then realised that the guidelines would follow the format of the structured record in the notes, and that the record itself might prompt referral, concealing the problem for the duration of the audit. A different method of collecting data is required, and after discussion it is decided that the rehabilitation staff should visit the ward to determine whether patients should have been referred. This approach is attractive because it is more likely to uncover the extent of the problem and could indicate a possible remedy. The audit may then generate evidence which could be used to persuade the service planners that this should become normal practice and that the necessary resources should be provided to achieve it.

The benefits of planning

The example of the audit of stroke patients showed that designing an audit study is not simply a matter of dealing in turn with a set of tasks; the decisions taken about one aspect of the study can have consequences for decisions previously taken. Thus although the steps in the design are given as a list and, although all need to be tackled, they will not necessarily be finalised in the order given. All aspects of the audit need to be considered before any one can be finalised, because all influence the study design.

The planning example also illustrates the scope for improvement in study design to be had from a consideration of all the stages of the audit *before* any data are collected. Health professionals usually know enough about their specialties, and where inadequacies of care are likely to lie, so that much of the planning can be achieved without data. However not all parts of the design can be developed without data. The exact nature of the health care problem, the reasons why it occurred and the most appropriate solution to it will often only emerge after data have been collected. Thus the development of audit studies needs to be undertaken in two phases: developing the initial design (without data); and evolving the detailed design (with data).

DEVELOPING THE INITIAL DESIGN

The activities which can be carried out before any data are collected are shown in Table 10.1. These are: getting the group together and identifying what could be audited; developing

Table 10.1   *Developing the initial design*

Preliminary planning
- Establish audit group
- List potential topics
- Select important topic
- Start small

The early design
- Describe specific area of care
- Develop standards (criterion, target and allowable exceptions)
- Explore possible methods
- Review strategies for change

Negotiate group agreement
- Ensure all relevant staff involved
- Agree importance of topic
- Discuss commitment to change

Write a preliminary protocol
- Assess whether group has necessary skills and resources

---

the early design; and then ensuring that the group really wants to carry out that study. The result of these early activities should be a preliminary protocol describing an outline study design.

Preliminary planning

Establishing the audit group is not simply a matter of getting together with a few colleagues. The group will need to address the real concerns which audit raises; emphasizing that the audit is under local control and that all findings are confidential (see Chapter 3). A list of potential topics can be generated through discussion and possibly literature review, from which specific ones for detailed assessment can be identified. The procedure for generating topics and identifying those of most importance was reviewed in Chapter 4.

At the start of an audit programme it can be useful to carry out small studies. These can be completed quickly, sometimes producing results within a few weeks of starting. Seeing how audit can describe and resolve deficiencies in health care helps to stimulate enthusiasm for audit. This may help to convince waverers that change can be beneficial, and need not undermine professional competence or reputation.

The early design

Once agreement on the importance of the area for audit is reached, the topic needs to be clarified. This will seldom be conducted as a single step, but is approached incrementally. An initial assessment can often be achieved without formal data collection; clinical experience or a brief literature review may be sufficient. Only if doubt remains about the existence of the problem should data be collected, and this should be limited to a preliminary exploration. These early activities should also consider the type of standard which could be used, deciding the appropriate criterion and the performance target to be attained (see Chapter 5).

The preliminary investigations and standard setting should indicate whether, at least at first sight, the project is worthwhile and practicable. They should also clarify the types of data to be collected and the method of audit to be used (see Chapter 6). One of the principal benefits of planning is the clarification of the types of data which are needed, preventing the collection of unnecessary data, and ensuring that the audit goes much further than simply observing current practice (the fate of too many recent audits).

The design of any study involves a compromise between what would be ideal and what can be achieved in practice. For example post-operative pain is a significant clinical problem which is not always adequately managed [3]. One area of compromise is the sample of patients included in the audit. The ideal would be to include all patients operated on, but inevitably some will be lost to the study, e.g. those discharged early or those too ill to complete a questionnaire. Similarly, because there is no objective measure for assessing pain, subjective measures, such as self-reported pain, or proxy measures like reported sleep loss would have to be used. The skill of study design is knowing when such problems are sufficiently important to threaten the validity of the study of knowing how quick and dirty is too quick and dirty. Thus patients discharged early are unlikely to be suffering more pain than those still in hospital and could be omitted without problem. In contrast being too ill to answer questions may in part be due to post-operative pain, so that omitting these patients could conceal the true extent of the problem.

The culmination of this early planning is a review of the possible strategies for effecting change. The intention is not to identify the appropriate strategy, but to assess whether this topic is likely to be amenable to change, and whether a consideration of the types of strategies which might be used could influence the study design.

Group agreement

When the initial design is formulated, all the professionals likely to be affected by the topic need to be identified and involved in the audit. For example the stroke study began with a geriatrician, junior doctors, and nurses, but was expanded to include the rehabilitation services. Successful preliminary planning should lead to agreement that the topic is worthwhile, that there is a good chance that the project is practicable, and that it can be conducted within the resources available. The intention is to reject projects which are clearly unimportant or impracticable as early as possible, to minimise the waste of resources. Agreement on the importance of the topic could lead to an early commitment from group members to a willingness to implement change should deficiencies in care emerge. Strategies for reaching consensus in groups are discussed in Chapter 3.

A preliminary protocol

A convenient way of clarifying the design is to write a protocol. *'Usually the plan in one's mind is not as clear and logical as was hoped, and the gaps and flaws are easier to recognise and correct when the plan is seen on paper'* [4]. The level of detail will depend on the study, but all the stages should be covered. Even when a group is not initially seeking outside funding, preparing a protocol is often a salutary experience. It forces attention to be given to the whole of the audit cycle and provides a focus for the critical assessment of the study.

A typical protocol would provide an introduction indicating why the audit is needed, giving a clear statement of its aims. It would describe all the features of the study design.

Individual tasks identified in the protocol can be delegated to individuals or small groups. This responsibility may help concentrate the minds of the named individuals on whether the audit is practicable, and whether there are sufficient resources to carry it out.

EVOLVING THE DETAILED DESIGN

Much of the planning can be achieved before any data are collected, clarifying the types and likely sources of the data which are needed. But to complete the design data will be required, in particular to identify the underlying causes of the problem and enable the appropriate solution to be developed. Data can influence the study design at several stages, leading it to evolve as shown in Table 10.2. Because data collection involves many technical considerations, such as sample size and sampling method, it is reviewed in a separate section.

Table 10.2 *The evolving design of an audit study*

Confirm problem exists

Reassess the design

Describe problem in detail
- Identify underlying causes of the problem
- Identify barriers to change
- Decide whether change required

Plan for change
- Confirm intention to implement change
- Develop strategy for change
- Implement strategy

Monitor the impact of change
- Assess impact of strategy
- Decide whether further action necessary

Confirm a health care problem exists

The initial role of data is to confirm that the problem is real and worth tackling. This will often involve only limited data collection, and is a preliminary step that allows the audit group to decide whether and in what ways further steps should be taken. Beginning the audit with a review of the findings from limited data collection emphasises that the members of the audit group are in control of the study.

Reassess the design

Whenever data are collected, the study design should be reassessed in the light of the findings. It is likely that several features of the design may need to be revised, especially to:

- Ensure all relevant staff are involved.
- Reassess importance of the topic.
- Agree standards.
- Select method.
- Outline detailed plans for data collection.
- Assess the skills and resources required.

The endpoint of these assessments should be a finalised version of the protocol which describes the study design for a detailed investigation of the problem.

Describe the problem in detail

Knowing that a problem is real is not necessarily the same as fully understanding it. The main stage of data collection is intended to yield that understanding and clarify the scale of the problem; identifying the underlying causes, and indicating the potential barriers to effecting change. This will enable a decision to be taken on whether change is required, and will indicate the strategies which may be successful in remedying the problem.

Plan for change

Strategies for change are more likely to be effective when developed by all the members of the audit group (see Chapter 8). Solutions imposed by others will often be resisted. Starting from an agreement that the problem is an important one, a tailored solution can be developed by the group. There are many possible approaches to effecting change. The one selected should be that which the group feels is best suited to remedying the underlying causes of the problem and overcoming the potential barriers to change.

Monitor the impact

Ensuring that the desired changes have occurred following the implementation of a strategy for change is the final stage of the audit cycle. It is often found that although some improvement in the delivery of care has occurred, further improvements could be made. Thus the assessment of current practice has to be repeated and a new decision taken on whether additional action is necessary.

DESIGNING THE DATA COLLECTION

The review of designing audit studies identified several points at which data are required. Whatever the purpose of the data, attention to some general rules will simplify their collection:

- Avoid premature data collection.
- Specify the data to be collected.
- Identify best source(s) of data.
- Design simple record form.
- Decide the methods of data processing.
- Prepare operations manual.
- Ensure confidentiality.
- Estimate appropriate sample size.
- Describe the method of sampling.
- Outline the principal analyses to be conducted.
- Construct a timetable.
- Conduct pilot study.

Premature data collection

One of the major pitfalls in audit is selecting a method and beginning data collection too soon. Data collection is the stage of audit which can consume most time and effort for least reward. It is often tempting to collect data with no clear purpose in the hope that this will provide insights, leading to the design of a more effective audit. Unfortunately early data collection exercises often achieve little; more can be achieved by careful thought than by filling cabinets with data. The alternative approach recommended in this book is that each step in the audit cycle should be considered first, and a plan including all the steps be drawn up before data collection is begun.

Specify data to be collected

The process of designing the audit study before beginning data collection should have clarified the exact purposes for which the data are required. A clear specification of purpose will help identify which data items are required and avoid the common problem of collecting items which are of little relevance to the audit in hand. As a general rule, all items which fall into the *'it might be interesting'* category are probably inessential (see Chapter 6 for a fuller review of the purposes of data).

Identify the best source of data

Data for audit can be obtained from a variety of sources in addition to case-notes, e.g. the pharmacy, pathology laboratory or coroners' reports (see Chapter 6). Often the same information will be available from more than one source, forcing a choice of which to use. This will be a compromise between ease of access and the accuracy and completeness of the data.

Construct the record form

The design of the record form or questionnaire follows when the data to be collected and the sources from which it is to be obtained have been decided. The form is arranged to facilitate the collection of accurate data and to minimise the effort of recording. The principles for the construction of record forms and questionnaires are reviewed in Chapter 7.

Describe the data processing method

Some audit studies may involve little more than identifying those patients who fail to meet the agreed level of care. For example an audit of the delay between referral and first consultation simply kept a list of patients on which the relevant dates were recorded (G Blamire, personal communication). However sufficient data will be collected in most studies such that processing by computer will be necessary. Various methods of data processing are described in Chapter 7.

Prepare an operations manual

For small studies which involve only a few patients or collect one or two items of data on each, it will be clear what has to be done and how it is to be done. However for larger studies, particularly those in which junior staff are delegated tasks, an operations manual can be useful. It specifies what data are to be collected, how measurements are to be made and on which patients. It should also indicate how the data are to be coded. The manual not only makes it easier to train staff to collect data of high quality, but can also help with the interpretation of the findings. It is remarkable how many study details, which were so clear at the time of data collection, become a faint blur after only a few months.

Ensure confidentiality

When planning the data collection, attention needs to be given to mechanisms to ensure confidentiality. Explicit recognition of this will often help allay the concerns of those intimidated by the thought of audit. Code numbers can be used to identify patients and health professionals, with the key to the code being locked in a secure place. This key, and where necessary the original data, can be destroyed when the data have served their purpose. Often this will be before the findings are circulated outside the audit group.

Estimate sample size

One of the main aims of good study design is to provide a good estimate of the proportion of patients who meet the criterion of good quality care (Chapter 5). However, because of the play of chance, the quality of care found in the sample of patients studied may differ from that of all patients treated. The size of an audit is chosen to reduce the effects of the play of chance to an acceptable level. The question of what is acceptable, and methods for calculating sample size, are reviewed in Chapters 6 and 9.

Choose sampling method

Sample size calculations sometimes indicate that there are more patients to hand than are needed, so that a method of selecting the desired number is required. The method may be simple, for example including all patients seen over a set time period such as six months, or it may be more complex, involving selecting a sub-group of patients. Whatever method is chosen the important point is that it should not lead to a sample of patients who are systematically different to all patients treated. For example if the outcome of hysterectomy were being audited, it would not be advisable to include only those patients discharged within one week of the operation. This would exclude many of the patients experiencing complications, because their stays would be extended. Methods of sampling are reviewed in Chapter 6.

Outline the analyses

Strictly speaking specifying the analyses to be conducted is not part of data collection. However doing so before collecting any data helps to ensure that:

- Essential data are collected.
- Design is fully worked out.
- Statistical expertise is available.

Possibly the worst outcome of an audit study is to discover at the end that the key piece of information to reveal why care was unsatisfactory was not collected. Collecting masses of information is no guarantee against this, but thinking through beforehand the analyses to be carried out can help. One useful technique is to draw up blank tables, labelling the rows and columns, in which the main findings of the study will be presented. The discipline of doing this will often suggest key factors, previously overlooked, which would be important for interpreting the findings.

As part of thinking through the analyses to be conducted, the likely sources and sizes of biases and errors in the data need to be considered. The idea is to decide whether these potential problems could be large enough to invalidate the interpretation of the study. If so the design may need to be modified to reduce the problems using the strategies reviewed in Chapter 7.

Construct a timetable

Constructing a timetable specifying when each phase of the data collection should be achieved provides an easy means of identifying unexpected delays. Data collection exercises frequently get bogged down; case-notes may be hard to trace, the workload may be much greater than expected, the design of a coding system for the data, or the development of the data processing system may be beyond the experience of the staff. Whatever the reason, the breakdown will only be detected speedily if progress is monitored regularly. Otherwise, particularly for studies which take several months to complete, no progress might be made for some weeks or months before this became apparent. The construction of a timetable can also help in assessing the resource requirements needed to complete the audit in an acceptable time, highlighting the feasibility of the study.

Pilot study

Before beginning data collection for real it is essential to carry out a pilot study to identify any defects in the design. Several features of the study need to be assessed, including making sure that:

- Staff are adequately trained.
- Relevant data are readily available.
- Sufficient patient numbers can be obtained.
- The resource needs are acceptable.
- The timescale is realistic.
- The instructions are clear.
- The form for data collection is easy to complete.
- Study design is appropriate.

When first developed most study designs contain flaws, which are best identified by trying them out. Resolving problems at an early stage not only prevents subsequent wringing of hands and gnashing of teeth, but makes it more likely that the audit will achieve its ultimate aim: improving patient care.

PREPARING A REPORT

The final stage of any study is the preparation of a report. There is no better way of ensuring that you really understand what was done and what the findings mean than writing them down for others to share. The report need not be lengthy; short and simple are to be preferred to long, complex and, in all probability, boring. But whatever the size it should usually follow a set structure, giving:

- Background to the health care problem.
- Aim of the study.
- Data collection methods.
- Source and number of patients.
- Findings, presented in tables and graphs.
- Discussion of the key findings.
- Actions taken to effect change.
- A decision whether further action is required.
- Assessment of the wider implications of the findings.

Preparing a report is not only for those who hope to publish the results in a professional journal. With the current emphasis on health professionals to be involved in audit, a report may be needed to show that it is being actively pursued. It will also show that the necessary steps to maintain high quality of health care are being taken. Ensuring high quality of care is the essence of audit. The circulation of reports on quality of care helps create the environment in which quality is improved from the good to the excellent.

REFERENCES

1. Abramson JH. Survey Methods in Community Medicine. London: Churchill Livingstone, 1990.
2. Hulley SB, Cummings SR. Designing Clinical Research. Baltimore: Williams and Wilkins, 1988.
3. Kuhn S, Cooke K, Collins M, Jones JM, Mucklow JC. Perceptions of pain relief after surgery. Br Med J 1990; 300: 1687–90.
4. Friedman GD. Primer of epidemiology. New York: McGraw-Hill, 1987.

Index

Index compiled by Geoffrey C. Jones